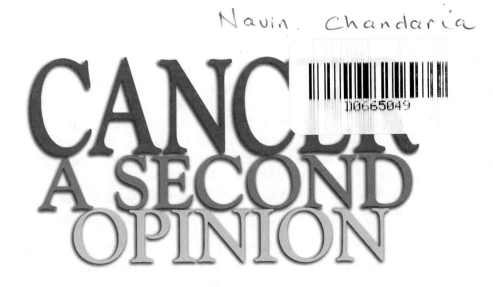

CANCER
A SECOND
OPINION

JOSEF ISSELS, MD

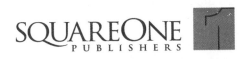

SQUAREONE
PUBLISHERS

The information and advice contained in this book are based upon the research and the personal and professional experiences of the author. They are not intended as a substitute for consulting with a health care professional. The publisher and author are not responsible for any adverse effects or consequences resulting from the use of any of the suggestions, preparations, or procedures discussed in this book. All matters pertaining to your physical health should be supervised by a health care professional. It is a sign of wisdom, not cowardice, to seek a second or third opinion.

For more information on the work of Josef M. Issels, MD, you can contact The Issels Foundation Inc. by calling toll free from the United States and Canada at 1-888-DR ISSELS, from other countries at 619-221-996. The Issels Foundation can be reached on the web at www.issels.com

Square One Publishers
115 Herricks Road
Garden City Park, NY 11040
(516) 535-2010 • (877) 900-BOOK
www.squareonepublishers.com

ISBN 0-7570-0279-X

Printed in the United States of America

10   9   8   7   6   5   4   3   2   1

Contents

Illustrations

Diagrams

To my dear wife

Ilse Maria

Foreword

FOR FORTY YEARS I ACCOMPANIED DR. JOSEF ISSELS on his "road less traveled" as his wife and collaborator. For forty years I have witnessed that "incurable" cancer patients can be cured through comprehensive immunotherapy and remain cancer free for decades. It is my sincere wish that many more cancer patients may benefit from the experiences presented in this book, and I thank Rudy Shur for helping get the word out by publishing this classic health edition.

Dr. Josef Issels' significant contribution to cancer medicine (and not *only* to cancer medicine) is recognized by many reputable researchers in this field. He was the first to integrate standard and alternative/complementary treatments into a comprehensive therapeutical concept within which each modality has its clearly defined task to fulfill.

In 1951, Dr. Issels was the first to found a hospital specializing in the treatment of conventionally incurable cancer patients, and subsequently treated more than 12,000 of these patients on an in-patient basis for months at a time. Daily clinical observation of similar advanced cancers led to new insights into the body's inherent regulatory, repair, and defense mechanisms, which he incorporated into his treatment system. Dr. Issels pursued research on immunological and microbial aspects of cancer etiology since 1948, and established several research units in his hospital from its inception. In 1970, the hospital grew from 85 to 120 patient beds, and expanded its extensive research facilities, including the microbiological, immunological, dental, and hyperthermia units. During the hospital's early years, Dr. Issels and his co-researchers developed cancer vaccines in the laboratories on the premises. From 1958 until 1973, Professor Franz Gerlach of the University of Vienna, Austria, researcher at the Pasteur Institute, and Fellow of the Academy of

Medicine in Paris, France, was director of research of the microbiological department of the Issels Hospital. It became the only institution of the era to conduct research on mycoplasma in cancer and chronic degenerative diseases. Recent research by reputable US scientists suggests a link between mycoplasma and cancer, as well as chronic degenerative diseases.

Since the late 1960s, all German insurance companies have covered the treatments given at Dr. Issels' hospital. In 1970, London's British Broadcasting Corporation aired a sixty-minute television documentary on Dr. Issels' work in its "Tomorrow's World Program." From 1981 until his retirement in 1987, Dr. Issels served as an expert member of the German Federal Government Commission in the "Fight Against Cancer." He authored over fifty papers and three monographs on his treatment for cancer and its results. Independent statistical studies have been published in peer-reviewed medical journals.

I am happy that our son, Dr. Christian N. Issels, follows his calling with the same dedication as he carries on his father's legacy. At the Issels Medical Centers, he and his team continue to integrate scientifically validated alternative/complementary and conventional methods to meet the unique requirements of individual patients and enable true healing.

ILSE MARIE ISSELS

Introduction

EVERY SECOND OF EVERY DAY, A MAN, WOMAN, OR CHILD DIES OF cancer.

That one statistic explains why I felt the need to write this book, for in spite of the billions spent on research; on the refinements of surgical techniques; on the development of more sophisticated radiation machines; on the search for a drug to eradicate every cancer cell in the body which does not produce side-effects so unpleasant as to limit severely the amounts prescribed; on the hunt for a steroid able to totally combat the hormone-related cancers; on perfecting a biological strategy to the point where it is always able to marshal the body's own natural defences into fighting malignant cells; in spite of all this, one out of every six persons alive today will contract, and die from, cancer.

The malignant, crab-like cullular malfunction, which began to multiply at bewildering speed in their body tissue, will for those countless millions, tragically bring the realisation that their cancer could not be cured, controlled, or even contained, by the usual methods of surgery, radiotherapy and chemotherapy. Four out of every five persons who receive one, or all, of these treatments die within five years. That is not only an indication of the destructive power of the disease, but also a sobering reflection on the limits of standard techniques, and the concepts of cancer on which they are based.

These methods have one common factor. They treat cancer *in loco*. The surgeon is primarily concerned with the excision of the *local* malignant tissue. Radiotherapy, to succeed at all, also depends on its ability to destroy cancer cells *in situ*. Both the surgeon and radiotherapist have always accepted there is no way of detecting whether a small number of cells have escaped beyond their *local*, original confines, spreading the disease, and so making it mostly incurable in terms of further operation or irradiation. Chemotherapy is then called into play in the hope that drug treatment will either eliminate, or reduce, the number of malignant cells which escaped. This too is very much a limited attack, and alas, one that with our present state of knowledge does not produce an encouraging record of long-term success. Much the same can be said for hormone treatment: the efficiency of steroids has not advanced much in the past thirty years; many oncologists have stopped using them.

The failure of these methods usually means the patient is left to die—unaware there is another proven and positive treatment still available, one that totally discounts the popular concept that cancer is a *local* disease. Because it involves the entire bodily defence systems, it is called *ganzheitstherapie*, or whole-body treatment.

The popular concept of cancer is that the disease is primarily a localised one; the hypothesis is that cancer cells and the ensuing tumour develop in what hitherto was a healthy body. Only when the tumour produces toxic effects on the organism does popular thinking recognise and accept cancer as a generalised illness, or "malignant disease"; this is particularly evident when secondaries have developed generally and the patient is cachectic. From this the *localistic* practitioners conclude the tumour must be regarded as the *cause* of the generalised malignant disease.

Whole-body therapists take a diametrically opposed view. Cancer is primarily a generalised disease, providing the substrate which allows the tumour to develop as the most important symptom, or sign. This means that a tumour can only develop in a diseased organism. Malignant disease therefore is the *cause* of malignant growth, whether the tumour is a primary or secondary one.

In short, those who believe cancer is a local disease think that the tumour comes first and only afterwards follows the generalised illness; those who think it is a generalised disease of the body believe that first comes the illness, and only afterwards the tumour. This is the crux of the matter—the fundamental point of divergence between the "localists" and the "whole-body therapists"—and from this basically different way of looking at cancer, they from then onwards take separate paths towards the solution to cancer.

All that follows in this book depends on a clear understanding of what I believe are two fundamental truths:

Cancer is a general disease of the whole body from the outset.

The tumour is a symptom of that illness.

Surgery, radiotherapy and the other standard tools, have, as we shall see, their place within the whole-body framework. But their role now becomes a carefully-tailored one, designed to meet the premise that cancer is not just a localised *affliction*, but a disease of the entire organism.

It is my contention, based on twenty-five years of clinical experience with over eight thousand cancer patients, that only by recognising the disease is, and always has been, one affecting the whole body from the outset, can it be more effectively arrested. By adopting that principle, the statistics of survival can be improved from the present grim position where eight out of every ten patients die having received all possible surgery, radiotherapy and chemotherapy. Many would undoubtedly have lived if their doctors had recognised some basic home-truths. They can be stated simply enough:

1. Cancer therapy will remain in a cul-de-sac as long as treatment is based upon a concept out-moded by the latest research. It is an unwritten law of medicine that the concept of pathogenesis, the origin of an illness, must form the basis of all treatment.
2. Surgery and radiotherapy are a necessary and important part of cancer therapy. But it must never be forgotten that on their own they cannot be expected to be the answer to a chronic systemic disorder. A symptomatic treatment can never be enough.
3. To be optimal a cancer treatment has to be a causal one.
4. Whole-body therapy offers a true causal treatment for every malignancy. It consists of a specific treatment against the tumour *while at the same time* offering a causal general treatment to restore the body's natural defence systems. This combined therapy offers lasting results.

My purpose in this book is to show, step-by-step, the theory and practice of how this can be achieved. It is designed as much for laymen as for doctors; its hope is to give a clear picture of a treatment which can also provide the so-called "incurable" with a real extension of valuable living, and even a cure.

Cancer, as those of us who work in the field know, has a language of its own; it is said with a great deal of truth, for instance, "that immunologists only speak to immunologists—and then not very clearly!" I have tried to avoid this pitfall by minimising the use of technical jargon. I hope that, by speaking plainly about it, the fear which so many people associate with cancer will be removed by the awareness that more *can* be done than is generally realised.

In a lifetime spent arguing the case for whole-body treatment, I have encountered much opposition and many misconceptions. My personal wish for this book is that it will clear away those misunderstandings, and with them the opposition, while at the same time encouraging other doctors to take up the challenge, and undoubted rewards in terms of patient survival, that this method of treating cancer offers.

I will not pretend that I have found it an easy path to have followed. But in the end all else is forgotten in the knowledge that here is a combination treatment which embraces also the skills of the surgeon, radiotherapist, chemotherapist, and immunotherapist, allowing them to co-operate, in a way never before possible, and in doing so, to save more lives.

THE ISSELS-KLINIK   JOSEF ISSELS
ROTTACH-EGERN
WEST GERMANY

1

To tell or not to tell?

CANCER, UNLIKE ALL OTHER ILLNESSES, CONTINUES TO MAINTAIN A widespread fear over people. There are definite moral, magical and retributive elements in the attitude of many usually sensible persons when they are confronted with a threat from the disease, either to themselves, or a loved one.

In spite of realistic health education programmes, especially in Britain and the United States, ignorance and old superstitions still prevail about what may cause cancer.

A recent survey in England revealed that one woman in five polled believed cancer is inherited, that it is contagious, like measles, or is caused by an immoral life-style. There are many Americans who believe the disease can be transmitted through tomato seeds, wearing tight girdles, using plastic utensils or aluminium pots. Certain scientific studies do claim that contact with plastic and aluminium utensils, *can*, under certain conditions, induce cancer. It is also thought that malignancies caused by virus-like organisms, *can*, in certain situations, be contagious. And, as we shall see a disposition to cancer *may* be inherited. Nevertheless, a well-entrenched back-log of folk-lore exists, colouring people's attitude to the actual manifestation of the disease. This follows a predictable pattern. A deep-rooted fatalism sets in. Resignation to the situation takes over. Cancer at that stage becomes synonymous with pain and death; it is something not to be discussed frankly, like heart conditions or a broken leg.

13

The belief that cancer is something not to be openly spoken about is too often fostered by doctors themselves whose own clinical experience in providing meaningful success in managing the disease has largely been disappointing.

They were taught, as I was, that to tell a cancer patient the truth can bring a loss of hope—because there was so little to offer. The modest advances in surgery, radiotherapy and chemotherapy, have not changed a widespread conviction these doctors have that there are some patients who simply do not wish to know the truth. That is understandable; for some patients it is probably enough to live from day to day. But often the decision to remain silent, or instead to tell a "white lie", is taken because the surgeon or radiotherapist cannot admit to their patients, or sometimes to themselves, that their methods are frequently only palliative and not curative.

Thus, an important factor in all successful treatment is denied to cancer sufferers because of a mistaken belief by the doctors that the truth is best ignored in all but a few special cases.

Sometimes this deception is maintained almost to the point of death, sustained by ever larger doses of pain-killing, mind-sapping drugs, that make it easier to pass off evasive answers.

Recently, a survey was carried out in a large hospital in Manchester, England, on patients who were told *after* treatment that they had cancer. Some found the knowledge uncomfortable. But seventy-five percent welcomed confirmation from their doctors of what they had suspected all along. They experienced a real relief that the "white lies" were over, that they could resume the "two-way partnership" which is the essence of all good doctor/patient relationships, and one which helps towards recuperation.

That survey prompts the question: how would those patients have reacted if they had been categorically told *before* treatment that they had cancer? I believe they would have used that knowledge to further a sensible attitude towards the illness.

Much of the superstition and fear in people's mind towards cancer can, I believe, be largely laid at the door of that still-powerful body of medical opinion which argues that the present state of conventional cancer treatment rarely justifies open honesty. They cannot altogether be blamed for their stand; statistically two out of every ten cancer patients only survive for five years or more after all possible conventional treatment has been tried; in such circumstances, argue these doctors, telling the truth can be cruel. In advancing this argument they are also implicitly admitting the limitations and failure of standard methods of controlling cancer.

For those doctors, the word "incurable" is never mentioned in a patient's hearing—no matter what suspicions may be harboured in the sufferer's mind. It is better, one distinguished specialist states, that his patients remain ignorant of their condition. It is a view many of his colleagues actively canvass support for.

It is one that I utterly reject on the grounds that a patient has the right to know the truth about his condition, and, more important, to know that he could be successfully treated when other methods have failed. It should be an accepted principle for every surgeon and radiotherapist who can do no more to correct the course of cancer, to explain the situation to his patients—and to place before them the possibilities of further beneficial help through whole-body treatment.

Knowledge alone does not, of course, conquer real, exaggerated, or imagined fears about cancer. Nor indeed does it play a direct part in the active treatment of the disease. But suspicion is a breeding ground for psychological stress—and that can affect the course of the illness.

It is a fundamental principle of my whole-body therapy that adult patients should be told the truth; because the treatment offers them a real chance, a new way, after other methods have failed.

This encourages patients to come to terms with the illness. I have clinically observed in the vast majority of my patients that being told the nature of their cancer has helped to instil a will to live. The patient knows the clinical picture, knows what must and can be done to improve it, and, having received the truth, is generally prepared to fight all the harder against his malignancy.

This two-handed partnership, building a bridge between doctor and patient over which the treatment regime crosses, is of vital importance. In such an atmosphere patients feel their fear of cancer diminishing and their will to survive returning—important factors in combating a disease which lowers bodily resistance and depresses the nervous system appreciably.

It is axiomatic at my clinic that, as far as possible, there are no secrets. Patients talk openly about their cancers. Peace of mind, engendered by knowing the truth, can help a diseased body. A lifetime of close clinical observation has completely confirmed for me the need for such an approach.

It is a sad fact that nearly all my patients show various degrees of stress, largely resulting from a realisation that conventional treatment, upon which they had placed such store, could not in their cases guarantee permanent relief.

Though they would not recognise it in such precise terms, they are imbued with a dangerous fatalism when they arrive at my clinic. This can only be alleviated with total honesty on the part of the medical staff.

The vital thing is to convince these patients, by word and deed, that medical science can offer more than the surgeon's knife or the radiotherapist's cobalt gun; that, important though they are, these weapons can be made even more effective when they are incorporated into the whole-body concept of treating the disease.

It is never easy to achieve this parity with patients who believe there is nothing left open to them. It can only be done by the doctor building up a meaningful contact with those he treats; hollow cheerfulness and stilted conversations have no part in this very demanding, but so worthwhile, facet of patient handling. Sympathetic and honest management of patients, providing them, and their relatives, with a proper flow of information must be always regarded as being almost as important as skilled help and the proper relief of pain.

By itself such an attitude cannot alleviate the physical symptoms. But what it does, and which should never be minimised, is to create a favourable climate in which those symptoms can be better attacked. The psychological state of many of these so-called incurables is almost immediately improved when it becomes clear to them that they are being actively treated, and are not just being left to die in a comfortable bed.

The question then, in whole-body therapy, is not *when* to tell, but *how* to tell the truth.

Firstly, there is a need for a carefully psychological assessment of the adult patient. Fear is a very necessary part of man's defence mechanism; after all it is fear that often makes a person become a patient in the first place. It is important to understand that fear, and gauge it in each patient before revealing the truth to him. Having done that the best step is to present the clinical symptoms as succinctly as possible.

This is not the time to hedge around with obscure terminology.

Having completed the clinical assessment, the patient is encouraged to ask questions. At first he may be reluctant to even mention the word "cancer". The doctor should recognise that this reaction is a sign that a more primitive force is at work rather than a patient's mere inability to come to terms with his situation.

Surveys, reinforced by years of observations of newly-admitted cases to my clinic, confirm that the word "cancer" has an evil connotation of its own. Therefore it is quite understandable that people are reluctant to use the word to identify their illness.

This attitude can only be overcome by the doctor speaking of cancer as just one more chronic illness which can be effectively treated by approaching it along the principles of whole-body treatment, while at the same time recognising the value of standard treatments. It is this combination, presented properly to the patient, which can help remove his fear, make "cancer" an acceptable word, and open the door to awareness that whole-body treatment is the best possible approach to the disease.

There is also a need for necessary caution over the inevitable question that all patients ask who are faced with the truth for the first time: that is the matter of hope in relation to a cure.

It has been said before, but deserves repeating, that this is a matter which needs the most careful thought from the doctor who decides to be frank with his cancer patients while at the same time offering them a genuine treatment outside that which is generally prescribed.

In 1956 I formulated a set of rules for my medical staff, putting into writing principles I had long adhered to. They are:

1. Never promise a cure to anybody.
2. In dealing with prognosis, tell a patient or his responsible relatives that the first step is to arrest the tumour.
3. That will prolong life.
4. The next step is to try and make the tumour regress.
5. That will bring a further prolonging of life.
6. The patient should be told that the eventual medical aim is to try and reach the stage where the tumour disappears completely.
7. Time itself is another factor. Patients should be told that cure *is* a matter of time—in their case five years free of disease, the statistical yardstick used to measure cure rates.

8. Our aim is to try and achieve that situation. But we can make no promises. And we never talk of "cure" but "remission".
9. We always talk with the knowledge that positive treatment can be offered. That is much more precise and beneficial.

By following those rules no doctor should fall under suspicion of offering false hope—a charge that is frequently levelled at those of us who argue more can be offered in the treatment of cancer than is generally available in conventional medical circles today.

There are some patients who cannot be told the truth: small children and those whose illness has rendered them unconscious. In these cases parents and relatives must be informed of the situation along the lines indicated.

In the case of children there is a special need to stimulate a strong doctor/parent relationship. Parents need support in the crisis they are involved with. This can only be achieved by real sympathy and a constant flow of information at each phase of the whole-body treatment. By working with, and through the parents, the doctor can then achieve the optimum effect for his young patient.

All relatives have a role to play in the clinical situation where doctors share the truth with their patients. Yet this factor is sometimes overlooked in the standard management of cancer. Too often relations are regarded as "not able to cope with things". In my experience the opposite is usually the case. From the outset of my clinical work I have always encouraged a policy of bringing relatives to the bedside of their loved ones, and, if needs be, to remain present even during a ward round.

In this way a patient does not feel divorced from the outside world, and the feeling that his cancer is a "special" kind of disease is diminished. The aim is to create a mood that in spite of the undoubted seriousness of the illness, practical treatment is still available, and that cancer must always be regarded as still being treatable after surgery, radiotherapy, and other standard techniques have failed.

None of this is possible without the right attitude from medical and nursing staff. Apart from proven professional skills, other attributes are essential to create an effective relationship with the cancer patient who is aware of his diagnosis.

Pessimism must never be allowed to take root. Gloom will inevitably rub off on to a patient, and his relatives, and could adversely affect the treatment regime.

The medical and nursing staff must always be encouraged to shape in the patient's mind a positive attitude towards cancer; the attitude must be towards total realism that cancer is not a bogey only treatable with surgery or radiotherapy.

The need for such an attitude is strikingly illustrated by a survey carried out among eight hundred British nurses. Questioned about the effectiveness of standard methods in the treatment of a number of cancers, their answers revealed a depressing but understandable view that little could be done.

This is one more reason for an urgent recognition that another method of treating the disease does exist, and that doctors are in a satisfactory position of being able to recommend this treatment in conjunction, where necessary, with surgery and other conventional means.

Having established such a framework of honesty, realism, and mutual co-operation, it then follows that cancer can be viewed less often as an incurable disease. This is not to oversimplify the problem: to do that would be as fatal as believing nothing more can be done when standard methods have failed. Nor must the beneficial effects of all such methods be lightly discounted. It is no part of my case that cancer is not cured by operations and X-ray treatments; it is my argument that, lamentably, such cures are not enough to warrant the very real misconception that they are the only answer.

The possibility of a total cure, by any definition, through standard methods, has not advanced significantly in the past forty years. Put another, and more realistic way, four out of every five patients failed to survive for five years after conventional treatment. In the 1960s there was high hope that this grim picture would improve with the advent of chemotherapy and hormone therapy. That promise, based on laboratory research, has still to be satisfactorily realised in the hospital ward. Hope had also run high that leukaemia and malignant lymphoma would be brought under control. That too has not been realised.

For even the most ardent well-wisher of standard methods, and I number myself among them, it is depressingly clear that the usual form of attack against cancer is still very much where it was a decade, and more, ago. There has been a great accumulation of knowledge about the *localised* tumour, but this is far from complete because it does not take into account the *general*, whole-body, nature of the disease.

In spite of the periodic bursts of optimism that fill the medical and lay Press, the situation will remain so until there is a radical rethinking among all oncologists about what cancer is. Painful though it may be, they must recognise that an impasse has been reached, and that it can only be overcome by a bold change of direction. Cancer scientists must turn away from a path they have followed, many of them for a working lifetime, and turn again to that older, and unassailable idea that cancer is a disease of the whole body. Only then can we progress; only then can we expect to see surgery and radiotherapy, and the other aids, play a more curative role as opposed to a palliative one. And perhaps only then will the "white lies" cease to be the stock in trade of so many doctors.

2

Cancer: The Multiple Enemy

CANCER IS INSIDIOUS, GENERALLY PAIN-FREE IN THE INITIAL STAGES, and frequently deadly by the time it is detectable. It has been described as savage cells which somehow evade the laws of the body, corrupt the forces which normally protect the body, invade the well-ordered society of cells that surround it, colonise distant areas, and as a finale to this cannibalistic orgy of flesh consuming flesh, commit suicide by destroying the host (McGrady).

What needs to be added to such an evocative description is that cancer is not one disease, but a word used generically for different, but related diseases; depending on the criteria applied to their classification, cancer is a word applied to one hundred and fifty and more, forms of the disease.

A more prosaic definition is that cancer is a disorder in which cells in the body multiply in a seemingly unchecked way, a proliferation in which they tend to lose or change their normal biochemical characteristics.

From that necessarily very general description—for scientists are deeply divided on even how to define cancer, given the present state of knowledge—spring a number of questions. What can be done about these renegade cells? How can they be inhibited from trespassing into healthy tissue? Why do they lie in wait for years, sometimes a quarter of a century, in an outwardly healthy body, before turning malignant?

The answer to all these questions is short: nobody really knows.

In 1806 a committee of respected American physicians posed important questions regarding such fundamental problems as an exact definition of cancer, identification of precancerous conditions, if any, and proof that cancer was either a contagious or hereditary disease.

The fact that many of those questions are still to be fully answered, some one hundred and seventy years later, is a chaste reminder of the complexity and magnitude of the cancer problem. Nor indeed is it one problem; a more accurate definition has been made by the English oncologist, Francis Roe, who speaks of "a galaxy of problems".

Roe's words underscore the fact that the present state of research into the nature and definition of cancer still leaves much to be resolved.

It is not my intention here to join in a generalised debate about the effects of the loss of cellular growth control; the reduction of a cell's power to differentiate; whether the cancer parasite transforms a healthy cell into a malignant one that cannot mature by differentiation; the effect of the removal of that little understood phenomenon known as cell contact inhibition; the function of enzymes in the complex micro-universe system of cells; the precise structure of chromosomes and the nature and extent of their activity; the workings of antigenicity, the body's capacity to elicit an immune response; all these functions, and the role they play in developing cancer, have still to be positively defined.

That situation will remain so until the essential differences in precise biochemical or physiochemical terms are resolved.

Much has been written elsewhere about the nature of the problems and attempts to overcome them; the published work on biochemical functions would completely fill a four-bedroomed house. I do not intend to add to such theorising, only to urge one fact. The whole problem of cancer in terms of growth, in terms of control, in terms of prolonged remission, turns on the bed-rock that the disease is one of the organism as a whole. This generalised condition provides the substrate in which the tumour is a symptom, albeit an important one. This means that a malignant tumour can *only* develop in a diseased organism.

In the past decade this truism has come to be recognised by clinical investigators, particularly in Britain and the United States. In recent immunology, promising belief has been explored that cancer is virus-induced which implies that the body has a natural resistance which plays an important role in cancer. This is borne out by the fact that disturbance of regulatory mechanisms and of functions, as well as of metabolism, are actually demonstrable *before* the tumour itself appears. Even these preliminary conclusions add weight to the argument that cancer can only be viewed, in terms of definition and management, as a disease of the whole body.

Reinforcement for this belief came at the Tenth International Cancer Congress at Houston in 1970. Scientist after scientist urged that to continue with present lines of research and treatment could only mean going from "crisis to catastrophe".

The Congress concluded that the possibilities of surgery, of radiology and of cytostatic chemotherapy have been largely exhausted and that no further worthwhile progress could be expected from such measures. This considered "second opinion" urged the need for the disease to be tackled from a fresh approach.

Some oncologists left Houston to look again at ideas which have been considered suspect for the past century under the influence of those who believed cancer was a local disease. Concepts of humoral pathology, the imbalance in the mixture of humours, or body fluids; incomplete detoxication; poor bodily drainage; and the need to support the natural healing powers of the body—these old, long forgotten concepts were looked at again, assessed, seen to be worthwhile, and given new names.

Today, the terminology has been updated to speak of restoring normal homoeostasis, restoring metabolic disorders and reactivating the defence mechanisms. But whatever the labelling, the thought behind this radical departure from what has been held sacred for a hundred years is clear: cancer is a whole-body disease.

It always has been so.

The earliest documents known to mention the occurrence and treatment of cancer are medical manuscripts of Chinese and Sumerian origin, from the third millennium B.C. Physicians then thought cancer was caused by the derangement of regulatory processes and tried to correct this with drugs and the use of acupuncture.

The ancient Indian medical compendia, the Ramajana and the Ayurveda (about 2,000 B.C.) recommended herbal remedies, red arsenic and minerals, used in a variety of combinations, for the treatment of cancer. Superficial tumours were cauterised with a red-hot iron.

Hippocrates (460–377 B.C.) is considered the founder of scientific medicine as practised in The West. He was one of the classical writers on humoral pathology and his work contains numerous references to the causes and treatment of cancer. In his writings we find malignant tumours referred to for the first time, as *karkinoma*. He argued that "separation of the humours" ("blood", "phlegm" and "bile") through toxins arising in the body—and particularly the production of "black bile"—were thought to cause disease. He recommended the detoxication of the body by means of suitable agents; surgical intervention should be used as a last resort. Arsenic, sulphur, laxatives, cantharis, hellebore, sandarac and other substances could be employed to treat cancer internally.

Hippocrates prescribed a special diet for patients. The Greek word *diaita* means "mode of life". It therefore refers not only to nutrition— as we have come to apply it in the narrower sense—but also suggests abstinence from anything that "might be deleterious to the mode of life in relation to the soul and spirit".

Hippocrates documents case histories describing the cure of cancer patients. His teaching, considerably extended by others later, remained the guiding principle in medicine until the eighteenth century.

Asclepiades (128–56 B.C.), a Greek physician living in Rome, argued that matter—including living matter—consisted of very small, indivisible particles, atoms, and could not be due merely to changes in humours, but rather it must be assumed that the "solid" parts of the organism were also involved. Asclepiades thus became the founder of "solidar", or structural, pathology. In spite of his atomistic views, he was not a "localist"; on the contrary, he was a "wholist", a general physician in the best sense of the word, attacking the use of powerful drugs and preferring natural methods of healing such as diet, herbal mixtures, physical exercise.

All told, Clarus Galen (A.D. 131–200), the founder of experimental physiology and pathology, wrote five hundred works, including various manuscripts on cancerology. Like Hippocrates, Galen adhered to the humoral doctrine. He considered "black bile", *atra bilis*, of particular importance, regarding it as the cause of cancer. This dogma remained, undisputed, into the eighteenth century. Galen also regarded cancer as a disease of the whole organism due to constitutional factors. In his opinion medical treatment should come first, with surgery playing a supportive role. He also gave very clear directions as to diet with his cancer therapy, listing foods that were forbidden and others permitted.

In the very early Middle Ages, Oribasius (A.D. 325–403), personal physician to the Emperor Julianus Apostata in Byzantium, wrote a medical encyclopaedia of seventy volumes. Causes of cancer were said to be "black bile" as well as a "fermenting substance" and "acridity of the humours". He stated that cancer was curable if one succeeded in eliminating the toxins from the organism by suitable measures.

Paul of Aegina (A.D. 625–690) stated that cancer might develop anywhere in the organism, internally or externally. Surgery he recommended only for breast cancer.

It is note-worthy that all these physicians found that, in their experience and observation, proper detoxication was most important with any chronic disease, including cancer. They had mastered the art of using different plant and mineral mixtures to treat the specific dyscrasia lying at the root of particular chronic disease. We would not be doing justice to their medicine, which was a true art, if we were to regard it as mere regulation of the bowels.

Arabian medicine adopted the medical knowledge of the classical physicians and extended it into chemical and plant pharmacotherapy. Again, general medical treatment and detoxication were considered of prime importance in the treatment of cancer. The *Canon Medicinae*, a work of a hundred volumes published by Avicenna (A.D. 980–1037) was still considered the best textbook of medicine at the time of Paracelsus.

Like Arabian medicine, the western pre-Renaissance "monastic medicine" aimed chiefly to improve on the materia medica of plant and mineral substances. A number of specific herbs were described which were said to "disperse" carcinomatous tumours. Surgical treatment was not used except when absolutely unavoidable. Even such eminent surgeons as Lanfranchi of Paris, whose *Chirurgia Magna* appeared in 1296, subscribed to this view.

Bombastus Theophrastus von Hohenheim (1493–1541), known as Paracelsus, the most outstanding physician of the new era then beginning, the great reformer of medicine, experimented with many of the formulae given by the Arabian alchemists and also used them, successfully, to treat cancer. He stated that "it is not the physician who heals, but nature". The physician should encourage nature's healing processes by suitable measures. Paracelsus therefore saw reinforcement of the body's own defence as an essential part of therapy. He said that with every disease one should "get to the bottom of it and discover its original cause".

Among the plant remedies which he used were the hellebore, one of the Ranunculaceae, which has medicinal actions similar to those of mistletoe; the crooked yellow stonecrop (Sedum); Arnica and other compositae, and also garlic, onions and wild leeks (Liliaceae). Minerals which he used were arsenic, sulphur and various mixtures of salts. The results which he obtained must have been impressive for Paracelsus wrote:

> It should be forbidden and severely punished to remove cancer by cutting, burning, cautery, and other fiendish tortures. It is from nature that the disease arises and from nature comes the cure, not from the physician. And so, with disease coming from nature, not the physician, and the remedy too coming from nature and again not from the physician, it must be the physician who must study both of these; and what they teach him, that must he do.

His system of treatment included not only remedies but also a form of psychotherapy, because the causes of every disease are "to be found in the soul and spirit as well as in the body". Paracelsus may therefore be regarded as the founder of the psychosomatic approach: "Let the highest motive in medicine be love."

Leonhard Fuchs (1501–1565), a professor at Ingolstadt, produced a detailed description of the efficacy of plant drugs in the treatment of cancer.

Ambroise Paré (1510–1590)—arguably the most gifted surgeon of the Renaissance—always expressed the view in his numerous books that cancer is a disease of the organism as a whole, and the treatment of the whole body should come first, before any surgical measures are indicated.

Johann Baptist van Helmont (1577–1644), professor at Leiden University, noted that psychic stress might lead to cancer, thus anticipating the discoveries of modern psychology by some three hundred years.

In 1650, René Descartes in France established the theory that "degenerated lymph" must be regarded the cause of cancer, as "black bile" could not be found anywhere. With this, the teaching of Galen's *atra bilis* as the cause of cancer, a theory which had persisted for more than a thousand years, was finally superseded. In Descartes's view, the malignancy of the disease is related to the condition of the lymph, and to its degeneration.

When in 1773 the question was put at the Lyons Academie: "What is cancer?", Bernard Peyrilhe won the prize with his answer which at that time was revolutionary: The cause of cancer could not be degenerated lymph, "but rather a toxin contained in this lymph", which Peyrilhe called "virus". At that time, virus meant merely "toxin", and not a micro-organism as we use the term today. This hypothetical virus was said not to be hereditary; only the disposition to cancer was inherited. Peyrilhe was the first to attempt to solve the problem of cancer and of secondary tumours by conducting animal experiments. His conclusion: "This disease is just as difficult to describe as it is to cure."

Georg Ernst Stahl (1660–1734), professor at Halle and Berlin Universities, returned to the theme of a recuperative power inherent in the organism. He called it the "anima". He regarded a raised temperature as one of the healing measures of the body and was against suppressing it.

Friedrich Hoffmann (1660–1742), professor at Halle and personal physician to the king of Prussia, used constitutional remedies in the treatment of cancer. He believed cancer to be hereditary, and gave a number of examples where the disease recurred in families.

John Hunter (1728–1793), professor of anatomy and surgery in London tried to give a new direction to the lymph theory. If Descartes's lymph was characterised by degeneration, Hunter's lymph was "coagulated", consisting of blood exuded from the vessels and becoming organised, being subject to biological laws. The real advance in this theory is that in Hunter's view "tumours arise because of activity of the organism itself; they are comparable to normal tissue, they live, grow, and are nourished by the organism." He stated that this lymph might also give rise to tumours which were not carcinomatous, but benign, and that more attention should be paid to the anatomical structure of tumours, to develop the art of diagnosis.

Hunter's aim was chiefly to understand the nature of cancer. Others were more concerned with the problems of therapy.

The system of treatment had essentially remained the same from antiquity to the new era. All the time, the aim had been to ameliorate the "acridity of the humours" in cancer patients by means of purges and other depurative, detoxicating measures, and also by dietary treatment. As to the tumour itself, chemical or plant remedies were applied externally or internally, to try and dissolve it, unless surgical intervention was possible—and indicated.

Arsenic had proved the most effective chemical agent. However, not infrequently it caused fatal poisoning, and because of this its inclusion among official preparations was continuously under dispute and at times even condemned. As a result, it tended to be very much an ingredient of secret nostrums.

W. R. Léfebure de Saint-Ildeford reported in 1775 that he had succeeded in curing cancer patients by giving arsenic internally. But his preparation of the drug was still very poisonous. In 1785, Thomas Fowler (1736–1801) finally succeeded in producing a formula for arsenic that was sufficiently effective and yet less toxic. This was called Fowler's solution and soon came to be generally used.

Another preparation taken from ancient days to treat cancer, both externally and internally, was corrosive sublimate and other mercurial preparations. These, too, were abandoned, because of their toxic effects, only to reappear again in secret nostrums. G. van Swieten (1700–1772), a pupil of Hermann Boerhaave (1668–1738), practising in Vienna, and his contemporary Sanchez (personal physician to the Empress Elizabeth of Russia from 1741–1761) recommended mercury for the treatment of cancer.

Other heavy metals have also been used internally and externally for cancer, among them copper, iron, barium, bismuth, lead, as well as silica and other minerals. Coal-tar, petroleum, turpentine, resins and many other natural products, and above all innumerable herbs, vulneraries and poisonous plants, were tried again and again in the treatment of cancer, right into the nineteenth century, with variable results.

While the treatment of cancer with chemical and plant products has always been subject to changing fashion, on the other hand the general constitutional treatment of the cancer patient, the fore-runner of whole-body therapy, has remained basically the same through the ages. It was generally assumed then, as now in whole-body therapy, that cancer was due to endogenous toxins in the organism as a whole. It was felt that in addition to local measures for treating the tumour, there was a need for purifying, detoxicating, consitutional agents, to change the patient's general condition. Implicit in all this was the concept that the cancer disease is a precondition for the development of the primary as well as the secondary growths; that the tumour was only a late stage symptom.

At the beginning of the nineteenth century, constitutional therapy was given new impetus by Samuel Hahnemann (1755–1843), the founder of homoeopathic medicine. Hahnemann argued that all diseases are basically due to a common cause, unknown internal toxins, which he called "psora". The psoriatic affection determined the constitution of the individual and his susceptibility to disease.

Persuasively, he contended medicine should be based on experience, on most careful observation of nature; the most important instruments in the treatment of disease are drug trials carried out by the physician on himself. With this, Hahnemann became the founder of exact, experimental pharmacology.

He arrived at the conclusion that the action of the drug used in any particular instance depended on the dosage employed. Given in high (subtoxic or toxic) doses, every drug caused an individual, specific syndrome of ill-health or poisoning. When low doses were given, the opposite effect was achieved. From this, Hahnemann deduced that it should be possible to use low doses of the remedy to remove the morbid symptoms produced by the very same agent given in toxic doses. This effect appeared to be all the more clearly demonstrable the more rarified the drug in question, so that its action became "potentised".

When Hahnemann and his followers systematically studied the drugs generally used in their day, they noticed that there were a number of substances which—given in toxic or subtoxic doses—could produce "tumours", cachectic states, and other signs of cancer. From this they concluded that conversely, highly attenuated preparations of those substances should prove beneficial in the treatment of cancer. They found that, in many cases, these remedies improved the syndrome, even resulting in some cases in the complete disappearance of symptoms.

More than a hundred years had to pass before "exact" scientific methods finally brought proof of the action of the small and indeed the very small dose. In plants and animals biologists have discovered active substances, for example the auxins, which evoke demonstrable reactions if present in quantities as small as the 0.0002 millionth part of a gramme —in homoeopathic terms the eleventh potency. Then there are the trace elements. In biological experiments on animals and plants many of them were found to have an effect in dilutions even higher than that. Kolisko obtained demonstrable variation in plant growth with dilutions in the thirtieth potency range. Many other homoeopathic preparations have since been investigated, in experiments in colloid chemistry, physics and biology. In every case the experiments have provided confirmation that even in very high dilutions—in "high potencies"—the substances tested produce objectively measurable effects (A. Bier, H. Wapler, H. Schoeler).

In 1883 Rudolf Arndt observed that the biological effect of a stimulus depends on its magnitude: weak stimuli excite the vital force, moderately strong ones favour it, strong ones inhibit it, and very strong ones arrest it. This phenomenon is known as Arndt's law.

Later Schulz, a German pharmacologist, drew attention to the analogy between Hahnemann's law of similars and Arndt's law. He carried out experimental studies and demonstrated that the fundamental law applies not only to physical but also to chemical, or medicinal, stimulation. It subsequently became known as the Arndt-Schulz law.

Perceptive physicians, gifted with intuition, and desiring to treat the patient as a whole, in addition to homoeopathy have long made therapeutic use of many other biological phenomena and methods of healing. They developed them further on an empirical basis long before "official" science took notice of such methods of treatment. Examples of this are acupuncture and electro-acupuncture. The advances made in modern, experimental medicine may be tremendous, yet, as Aschner put it, with some resignation, "we use barely a tenth of the effective methods of healing that are available."

For a thousand and more years, until the middle of the nineteenth century, generation after generation of physicians expressed the view that in the light of experience and observation, cancer must be considered to be due to constitutional changes, to a certain disposition, to functional and regulatory disorder, to a "decomposition of humours"—like all chronic diseases. Cancer, they said, arose through a complex disorder of metabolism and at the same time an inability of the body to eliminate the toxins which constantly develop. Whichever factor the prevailing theory made pre-eminent—bile, acrid humours, lymph, or some form of functional disorder—all agreed in one respect: that cancer was due to systemic disease and that the tumour was merely a symptom of that disease.

This concept comes surprisingly close to the latest present-day views on cancer.

The pattern of development of the disease was observed and described in detail by those past physicians and today we can confirm the validity of their observations when we treat cancer medically.

Did those methods used by the physicians of a bygone era actually prove effective against cancer? There is still a tendency today to deny this. Some scientists working in "modern" medicine believe they must refute and even ridicule those old-fashioned approaches to treatment. But they have themselves adopted quite a number of those empirical methods and have only attached a more scientific-sounding label to them: psychotherapy, hydrotherapy, balneotherapy, klimato-therapy, heliotherapy, dietetics, manualtherapy, physiotherapy and eliminative procedures such as venesection, leeches, pyretotherapy, purging, and fasting.

Yet in many respects the thinking of those old physicians does seem strange. Many reported cures do not exactly sound credible. There can be no doubt that at that time, too, possibilities of curing cancer were limited and unsatisfactory. But do we have the right to cast doubt on detailed reports describing successful cures of cancer in earlier times, or even to disregard them completely?

Surgical techniques were not so far developed at that time, and with no asepsis and anaesthesia it was obviously only possible to remove tumours that were easily accessible. The very effective local treatment that can be given today was indeed unthinkable in those days. However, the treatment of the patient as a whole, causal therapy aimed at the underlaying disorder, was much more fully developed and this side of treatment has not really been given adequate attention in the modern approaches to cancer therapy.

To sum up, we may say that until the middle of the nineteenth century medical thinking was governed by the humoral pathology of Hippocrates, of Galen, and of Paracelsus. In the medical histories and text books of those old physicians, one can always discern the clear thread of the idea that cancer is based on a general disorder. Following the unwritten law of medicine—the concept of an illness dictates its treatment—these doctors treated cancer for thousands of years as a general disorder. Thus their treatment of cancer was primarily medical.

But that was to change.

3

The Classic Methods

THE CHANGE IN DIRECTION AS TO WHAT CANCER IS AND HOW IT SHOULD be managed began some two hundred years ago. Unlike other revolutions, this was a quiet one, conducted in laboratories around Europe. The first hint of change came with the pathologist G. B. Morgagni (1682–1772). On the basis of earlier research and from his own findings from sections—the final stage of the illness—he concluded:

The seat and the cause of disease is in the organ showing pathological change.

This was the first step in pinpointing diseases, including cancer, as a localised phenomenon. The approach was furthered by histological examination.

Impetus to Morgagni's theory was provided by the French researcher, Xavier Bichat (1771–1802). He considered all tumours, benign or malignant, to have their seat in the connective tissue. His most famous protégé, R. Laénnec (1781–1826) developed this idea and published a text-book on the classification of malignant tumours.

One important fact emerges from the findings of those scientists:

The search for the cause of cancer was increasingly neglected as attention was focussed on the morphological structure and the classification of cancer.

But the limitations of the microscope, although invented at the end of the sixteenth century, meant only the macroscopic structure of cancers was accessible to researchers of that period. It was not until 1824, when Chevalier constructed the first achromatic microscope, that it finally became feasible to study cellular structures, allowing for a clear distinction between the cell, the nucleus and the nucleolus, and so creating the principle of cell formation. This also allowed for a distinction between normal and abnormal cells.

Johannes Mueller (1801–1858), one of the leading physicians of nineteenth-century Europe, succeeded in studying the fine structure of tumours under the microscope, pioneering work which showed that tumours also consisted of cells. Mueller was a physiologist, familiar with humoral pathology, and he felt that his findings only complemented what was already scientifically known. He, too, subscribed to the theory of "crasis", in which cancer is a disease of the organism and the tumour a symptom.

Then Rudolf Virchow (1821–1902), probably the outstanding figure in nineteenth-century pathology, established that cells multiply from existing cells and that connective tissue is the substrate on which all malignant tumours develop.

It was a brilliant and persuasive piece of original research. In 1858 it was followed by an even more outstanding work—Virchow's theory on cellular pathology, whose essentials were encompassed in the doctrine that all morbid processes occur in the cell. It laid the foundation stone for cellular pathology as we know it today. It also finally convinced the medical profession that cancer is a localised disease of the organism.

And yet a study of Virchow's writings shows only too clearly that in spite of his views on cellular pathology he still adhered to the belief that the organism should be regarded as a whole; he knew that his theory was a valuable one, complementing the existing ideas on humoral and neuropathology. But Virchow was the first to recognise that his doctrine did not supersede the older schools:

> Let it be emphasised once more that we fully acknowledge blood and nerves to be factors of equal significance to other parts, and that indeed we are in no doubt whatsoever as to their paramount significance, though we would argue that their effect is merely one of stimulation, of moderation, on other parts, and is not absolute.

Virchow clearly intended that his theory should be integrated with other pathological systems. When stating his views on the origins of tumours, he mentioned three factors which he considered particularly important:

1. The local situation.
2. A predisposition to disease based on the individual's constitution.
3. Dyscrasia, a malcondition of the body liquids.

In his three volumes on morbid tumours he wrote:
> If a specific change occurs in the blood and if there is also a pre-
> disposed site in the body, then the morbid blood will have a point of
> attack in that predisposed site—and give rise to disease.

Virchow's views on constitution were equally specific:
> In the organism, growth and development are generally determined
> by the type, and this type also determines the growth and develop-
> ment of tumours.

On dyscrasia he wrote:
> I myself do not hesitate to concede that it is necessary, considering
> the present state of knowledge, to ascribe the origin of some tumours
> to the blood, so that the basic disorder would be a dyscrasia.

It is clear from these passages that Rudolf Virchow, in spite of his
exciting discovery, still believed in disease of the entire organism. His
views on dyscrasia echoed those of Hippocrates, who taught that
dyscrasia was the basis for all kinds of diseases, which manifested themselves according to the constitution and disposition of the individual
person. Thus one patient has chronic rheumatism, another diabetes, a
third asthma, and a fourth cancer. So, from that, it can be seen that
cancer is not a unique disease. It is nothing more than another chronic
sickness.

And yet it is easy to understand now why this was overlooked.
Virshow's discovery made it possible to demonstrate beyond doubt
the morbid changes of disease in cells and tissues. It was a tremendous
event in an age when medicine was deeply concerned with presenting
a more "scientific image".

Virchow's work was eagerly seized as an opportunity to branch into
new fields. His findings were tangible, concrete evidence of a new
pathological process to be followed. The discovery was too recent as
yet for the medical world to realise that while it represented a pioneering
advance in diagnosis, it did not explain functional pathology. The

result was that humoral pathology—which does not only reveal how cellular changes have occurred but also co-ordinates the ground-rules for treating such changes—was set aside and cellular pathology adopted as a new "philosophy", rather than finding its rightful place within the existing framework of pathology. As so often happens during and after revolutions, under the tremendous impression of something new, doctors forgot what had been good in the old; the concept of cancer as a systemic *disease* faded into oblivion; research and treatment became focussed on the *tumour*. From a chronic disease of the whole organism cancer had become a local condition. The symptom of a disease was declared to be the disease.

This heralded a departure from a proven approach which physicians had followed for almost five thousand years. With attention focussed to such an extent on what went on in the cell, the concept of humoral pathology became neglected; the origins of the disease process were lost. Instead, a mechanistic view developed, seeing the disease as organic. That situation is still largely unchanged today, and I tend to hold it responsible for the present state of cancer treatment. While cancer therapy had previously been carried out at two levels—causally and symptomatically—it became, after cellular pathology had gained favour, the province of the surgeon.

The nineteenth century saw great advances in surgery, culminating in today's sophisticated surgical and anaesthetic techniques, resuscitation and post-operative intensive care which combine to make surgery relatively safe. Organic, vascular and brain surgery have been brought to high perfection by great men of medicine; in recent years spectacular organ transplantation has shown that the limits imposed on the surgeon are physiological rather than anatomical.

In this climate, where the barriers of surgical advances are breached in the full glare of the media, the optimism of surgeons understandably blossoms. Nowhere is this euphoria more evident than in some of the attitudes expressed towards the role of surgery in the management of cancer. If it is possible to remove the tumour radically, some surgeons believe, the body "can be rid of the disease from one hour to the next and made as fit as it had been originally" (K. H. Bauer).

Professor K. H. Bauer, a distinguished surgeon, a powerful advocate for the localised concept of cancer, and *ipso-facto*, a determined opponent of the whole-body approach, in 1963 restated the surgeon's creed as:

Sufficient reason for the surgical removal of cancer is given in the rates of cure through surgery, and because it has also been demonstrated experimentally that at least primarily and for a prolonged period cancer must be regarded as a local condition, or, to put it the other way round, that cancer absolutely never is a systemic disease. It is most surprising that there have actually been surgeons who subscribed to this notion, that cancer is a systemic disease.

One needs to balance that statement against the opinion of another equally respected surgeon, Sir John Bruce, Regius Professor of Clinical Surgery, Edinburgh University, Past President of The Royal College of Surgeons. In 1970 he expressed the view:

The future (of cancer treatment) lies elsewhere than in the operating room; but when the answer is eventually found, the surgeon will have no cause to be ashamed of his attempts to relieve suffering and not infrequently avert the arrows of death in one of the greatest scourges of mankind.

Of the two views, Bruce's words, I believe, offer a more realistic appraisal of the surgeon's role.

None of this is to minimise the functions of surgery as a treatment weapon: indeed, until quite recently it was the only method available in the conventional armamentarium for treating cancer. Surgeons have striven boldly and bravely in the hope that the physical destruction of growths and excrescences will bring lasting relief. They deserve credit for their surgical endeavours, and understanding for so often having to face failure.

I know from my own early experience as a surgeon that it is never easy to advise for or against an operation in known malignancy; the surgeon always balances the risk of operation with its possible mutilation against the consequences of leaving the tumour to probably cause the patient's death.

Having opted for surgery, the surgeon calls into play all his considerable skills and judgements only too often to see his efforts end in failure: for instance, only five percent of lung cancer patients survive for five years after surgery; eighty percent die within a year after such radical operations.

Faced with such depressing statistics, a further burden has been placed upon the cancer surgeon by the argument that the only way "to make sure" about the tumour is to carry out even more excessive ablation at the earliest possible stage—such as removing the entire stomach in early gastric cancer. In such cases the surgeon is faced with the question: should he, in effect, perform ever larger operations on smaller tumours?

Many feel impelled to say yes in the hope of effecting a complete cure.

Such thinking has led to the "primary super radical operation". In this kind of surgery the bladder and rectum may be excised; or, say, in the case of breast cancer, an arm and collar-bone as well as the Breast is removed. The views of Sir John Bruce will, perhaps, help the reader place this sort of surgery in context:

> There is no great scope for this sort of surgery, perhaps; but it must be conceded to have an occasional place in the curative repertoire of surgery. It is wrong to reject the concept of "super radical" surgery through ignorance of its possibilities, or repugnance to practise it. It demands of the surgeon courage, possibly humane ruthlessness, and certainly technical virtuosity of a high order. Its most important practical application is when disease has extended from its original site to involve organs and tissues in its immediate vicinity without having yet spread to more distant areas.

However, surgery continues to be powerless in one particular respect. Cancer is an insidious disease. Two-thirds of malignant tumours have already produced secondaries by the time a diagnosis is made, or they have infiltrated other structures around them to such an extent that surgery can offer no prospects of success. New developments in early diagnosis have brought little change in this situation. In such cases the surgeon is powerless, the patient inoperable, the prognosis incurable. Often the surgeon has also to realise that even the most careful radical surgery will not arrest the development of secondary tumours or recurrences in the original site. So more and more extensive surgery is performed. One example will show exactly the limitations of such extensive surgical intervention.

A woman of forty was diagnosed in a famous American hospital with a breast malignancy. Surgery was recommended and the entire breast was removed along with all the glands in the armpit. After a short rest period her ovaries were removed because the surgeon thought the breast cancer might be "estrogen dependent", that the hormones in her ovaries might have an effect on the residual tissues. Later he advised her to have a third operation, this time to have her adrenal glands removed to combat the progressive cancer that a series of radiotherapy and chemotherapy had failed to halt.

After the adrenalectomy, the surgeon advised her to have her pituitary gland removed; the pituitary is a small gland at the base of the skull regulating the functions of other hormone glands in the body. The woman did not recover from that operation, her fourth in a year. These were surgical attempts to find a surgical solution to a problem which was systemic.

It has been said, and the more enlightened surgeons accept the argument, that surgery in cases of cancer can often be no more than a cruel necessity. It is because of this that radiology has been embraced as an additional necessity and sometimes as an alternative to the scalpel. It seems less cruel; no flesh is cut; no blood is shed. But, in the view of one authority, "living tissue is destroyed, and the quiet dreamlike process, in which nothing of significance seems to happen, can eventually prove to be as painful and as dangerous as surgery".

A plea for acceptance of this situation has once more been recently advanced, this time by the radiotherapist Erich Easson, Chairman of the Commission on Cancer Control of the International Union Against Cancer. Easson argues, with some force, that, as with surgery, a temporary morbidity is an acceptable consequence of radiotherapy, to be tolerated as the price for success. He catalogues some of the side-effects: a radiation reaction in the organ or tissue treated, such as an "inflamed" throat with discomfort in swallowing; an inflamed bladder with frequent passing of scalding urine; diarrhoea following bowel irradiation.

Easson views these symptoms as no more troublesome than the after-effects of surgery and should be accepted as such; he also maintains that radiotherapy patients can be helped by "explaining away the mystique of the invisible rays, for some so-called radiation sickness is undoubtedly psychogenic and based on fear of the unknown".

It would be difficult, if not impossible, to explain to some patients that the permanent effects on their bodies were psychologically induced. Over the years I have seen many patients whose skin became brawny, thick, purplish, resembling the after effects of a severe burn from the ionising rays. Worse, the furrowed deep red patches on their skin too frequently had been inflicted in vain; the malignant cells had spread beyond the original irradiated area, so rendering the treatment virtually ineffective.

What are these rays? How do they work? What therapeutically useful biological effects do they create? How are these effects applied at a clinical level in man?

Some of the answers are straightforward enough; others cause intense debate even among the most committed radiotherapists.

In 1896 W. K. Roentgen read his classic paper announcing the discovery of X-rays. In the same year the French physicist Becquerel discovered radio-active properties in uranium. Pierre and Marie Curie then isolated radium and the other radio-active constituents of uranium.

By 1900 X-rays were being used to reveal bone fractures and other abnormalities, heralding-in diagnostic radiology. At around the same time came the realisation that X-rays and radiation could be used to provide new and undreamed-of methods of treatment. A year after Roentgen's original discovery it was reported X-rays would even make it possible to achieve the regression of malignant tumours.

Within a decade X-rays and the gamma rays from radium were found to have profound biological effects, the most important of which was their inhibiting effect on any growing or active tissue, such as normal blood-forming marrow. By 1910 this form of treatment had been formalised into radiotherapy, the treatment of mainly malignant disease by certain penetrating radiations. They became known collectively as ionising radiations because one of the effects they produce on passing through matter of any kind, including gases, is to split off electrons from their parent atoms, so producing highly reactive ions.

The early tubes used for radiation therapeutics were crude and largely ineffective. Then, in the 1930s came the realisation that the biological effects of X-rays and of gamma rays were similar and should be explored and developed together.

The production of more sophisticated X-ray tubes assisted this development. Then came a further major step forward—the recognition that radiation should be administered in a precise measurement or dose, just like any other drug. This measure became known as the Roentgen unit, a clinical yardstick indicating how much ionising radiation is necessary to create the desired biological effect. This laid the foundation for "modern" radiotherapy, with its wide range of machines capable of generating an energy of over ten million volts, with its linear accelerators and betatrons, producing finely focussed beams of electrons. As well as these "beam" machines, the discipline relies upon a wide range of radio-active isotopes or radium and radium substitutes, such as radio-active cobalt, gold, yttrium, tantalum. They all have their own special biological uses.

In using his equipment the radiotherapist needs great technical precision, for ionising radiations have the capacity to damage all living cells, healthy or malignant; the curative effect of radiotherapy is based on mutation leading to destruction of the nucleus of the cancer cell.

It is now generally accepted that radiotherapy gives the best results when used on superficial tumours. In cases like this, cancer of the skin for example, the therapeutic radiation dose is fully utilised for treatment, and does not damage healthy tissue; up to ninety-eight percent of all malignancies of the skin and lip can be cured by radiotherapy. Again, irradiation can also produce a temporary regression when there is secondary tumour growth, and in some cases it can even produce a permanent cure.

But the limitations of radiotherapy as a curative weapon have again been clearly defined: the curability of any cancer depends primarily on its dimensions at the time of treatment. A very large mass of cancer is unlikely to respond permanently to radiotherapy, "and even a small primary is incurable by available therapy, if the tumour has already shed secondary deposits via the blood stream to more remote parts of the body." (Easson)

In effect then, radiotherapy is a strictly locally effective weapon.

Nevertheless, and in spite of the technical skills of the radiotherapist and his technicians, the ionising rays, as we have seen, will frequently damage healthy tissue around the irradiated site. This can, and often does, have serious consequences for the patient, sometimes long after the course of treatment is completed.

Respected American scientists, such as Toolan and Murphy-Sturm, have demonstrated with animals that intensive radiotherapy damages the mesenchyme, the body's soft connective tissue, so depriving the body of its natural resistance. Patients who have received intensive radiation do not easily respond to immunotherapy or to treatments designed to activate natural resistance; it can take months to overcome this situation—a lengthy wait in cases where the time factor is critical.

Radiotherapy *has* played its part in the management, and even cure, of cancer, sometimes in inoperable patients. However, the last decades have confirmed that even the most advanced "beam" machines cannot always prevent the development of secondaries. The great hope that all cancers would be helped by radiotherapy has not been realised.

In the early 1970s the use of fast neutrons has given cause for hope that radiology might achieve more. Fast neutrons, unlike X- and gamma rays are less dependent for their effectiveness on the presence of oxygen in the tissue or tumour cells. But it may not be until the 1980s that their possibilities are clinically realised. Even then, radiotherapy will still depend on its ability to destroy cancer cells, to be, with surgery, a favourite weapon of the *localistic* theorists.

When surgery and radiotherapy have failed, chemotherapy is called upon to halt, if not to cure, the progressing cancer by the use of specific cytostatic or chemotherapeutic agents. However, the treatment of cancer only by drugs cannot yet produce a general cure except for a few rare tumours. In the overwhelming majority of cancers, the use of chemotherapy is still largely confined to inoperable, incurable, disseminated cancers. Nor are current drugs able to destroy every cancer cell in the body. Again, their side effects are so marked as to limit severely the amounts prescribed. That is the considered view of a proponent of drug therapy, Dr. John Q. Matthias, consultant physician at the Royal Marsden Hospital, London. It is one that few oncologists would dispute.

Chemotherapy, as such, is not new; for centuries doctors have used various chemical properties which are not poisonous to man, but toxic to an infecting organism, either destroying the parasites or stopping them from multiplying. Malaria, amoebic dysentery and many other infections have been successfully managed by the use of chemical agents derived from natural sources, such as chichona bark or the ipecacuanha root. The advent of penicillin and other antibiotics in the past few decades has made chemotherapy an exact science where striking success has been seen in many treatment areas.

And, despite the very necessary caution expressed by men like Dr. Mattias, it is satisfying to know that the search for suitable anti-cancer agents has produced some effective, short-term results from substances which inhibit the growth and division of cells.

Mitotic poisons have been developed which suppress cellular division; they include Trypaflavine, Colchicine, Vinblastine and

Podophyllin, all effective agents to combat mitosis, the process when the cell nucleus and its surrounding cytoplasm are about to divide. Other agents—among them urethene and nitrogen mustard derivatives (popularly known as Endoxana)—affect the resting nucleus, inhibiting the process during the resting phase between stages of active cell division; these are known as interphase toxins. The anti-metabolites are a group of substances which interfere with the formation of nucleo-tides and prevent the synthesis of nucleic acids, the extra RNA or DNA needed to ensure cell division takes place. These agents include the purine analogues, such as Puri-nethol, and the folic acid analogues, like Aminopterin. A number of antibiotics are used in the treatment of cancer, especially the actinomycins.

These cytostatic agents are used singly or in combination to destroy tumour cells circulating freely in the blood and lymph stream in an attempt to stop recurrences or secondaries. When these agents are used for follow-up treatment after surgery and irradiation, the risk of metast-ases has often been reduced; over the years it has even become possible to inhibit the growth of solid tumours and reduce them in size. Cyto-static therapy has also brought definite improvement in the results of treating systemic malignancies, particularly Hodgkin's disease and acute and chronic leukaemia in children.

Unfortunately it has been found that these agents are not selective; they interfere with the growth of normal as well as of cancer cells. All rapidly growing tissues, particularly the mucous membranes and hair follicles, suffer considerable damage with chemotherapy. It seems that in many cases the growth of healthy cells is inhibited more than that of the cancer cells. Because of this, cytostatics can only be used for limited periods. Nevertheless, chemotherapy has proved very valuable if carefully-measured doses are given on a short-term basis with rapidly growing tumours.

Long-term cytotoxic treatment still presents a problem with the present state of drug knowledge, because immunodepression may develop, seriously affecting the natural resistance of the body. Another problem still to be overcome is that malignant cells cease to respond to cytostatic agents after a time.

Interval therapy—a method by which patients receive one or two large doses, spaced at a span of two to three weeks—has proved to be more effective than smaller doses given every day. An example is the use of the cyclophosphamide Endoxana. The drug itself is unusual among chemotherapeutic agents in that the side-effects associated with its use are predictable and in almost all cases reversible. All the same they are drastic: alopecia, haemorrhage cystitis, nausea and vomiting, diarrhoea, mental depression, impotence and dermatitis are listed as possible side-effects. But giving the drug at wider-spaced intervals than usual does not impair the body's immunological mechanism in the same way as prescribing regular smaller doses of the drug.

In many cases interval therapy arrests further growth of the tumour and even achieves temporary regression. While tumour growth will usually start again after some weeks, interval therapy allows time to be gained, especially in the management of rapidly developing, incurable cancers, and during this time, as we shall see, immunotherapy may play a decisive part.

The problem complicating the search for totally effective anti-cancer drugs has been summed up in a report of an expert committee formed by the World Health Organisation to investigate the question. They considered that tumour chemotherapy is faced with a task of colossal difficulty, since it must learn how to destroy all the cells of each of an enormous number of varities of tumour, and, at the same time, avoid irreparable damage to any of the essential normal tissues, from which tumour tissues differ, in the main, only quantitatively. In these circumstances the success that has nevertheless been gained in discovering compounds that have a selective effect on some tumours—that may indeed bring about more or less complete regression of some animal and human tumours—must in itself be classed as a great achievement.

Those findings were made in 1962. Ten years later the state of cancer chemotherapy still remained uncertain as the ultimate weapon to eradicate the disease.

The arrival of the birth control Pill has made almost everybody aware of how hormones affect the human body. The Pill is the result of the manipulation of the ovary, the hormonal gland which produces the human egg; the Pill, a combination of either natural or synthetic hormones, prevents fertilisation.

Hormones, and there are about forty in all, are the body's chemical "messengers", synthesized in specialised tissues, such as the ovaries, testes, adrenal glands, pancreas and the pituitary. And long before the Pill became universally popular, hormones had been harnessed to treat certain types of malignancy, such as cancer of the breast or prostate. Male hormones are used on female patients and vice-versa. Given in extremely high doses they cause "hormonal castration" by suppressing the production and biological action of the female or male hormones normally produced by the diencephalo-hypophyseal system and the sex glands while at the same time inhibiting the process of malignant growth dependent on these hormones. These "opposite sex hormones" arrest tumour growth selectively, and do not affect normal cell growth, such as the formation of healthy blood cells, the way other cytostatic agents do.

Hormones have to be taken for several years regularly and without interruption, and in many cases over such a prolonged period they lose their potency to prevent the development of metastases. There is also another serious complication: the long-term use of hormonal treatment in high dosage causes personality problems; men become feminised while women acquire masculine characteristics, a situation that frequently causes psychological ravages almost as great as the physical destruction produced by cancer.

By themselves neither chemotherapy nor hormone treatments will ever be able to replace systemic medical therapy designed to eliminate the causes of cancer. Both should only be used as part of a logistical regime, and even then their use should be strictly limited to those cases where biological methods on their own will not achieve the desired results.

Enzyme therapy is another form of treatment which is also directed towards the tumour. It is based on the principle that foreign protein is "digested" in the blood and tissues just as the protein from meat or cheese is digested in the stomach (Abderhalden). For every foreign protein entering the organism, the body forms a specific enzyme which will digest only this one protein. The body is also able to remove any of its own cells which have become diseased by producing enzymes directed specifically against them. In the healthy organism, "cancer cell-digesting" enzymes are always mobilised as soon as a cancer cell develops anywhere.

Observation has shown that cells which have undergone pathological changes, through inflammation or through cancer, are also digested by non-specific, "normal" pancreatic and gastric enzymes. If cells are completely healthy, they resist attack even from concentrated enzymes.

But the enzymes are able to attack cancer cells because their enclosing cell membrane is far less strong than that of a normal cell. During cell division, the pores of this membrane are enlarged to such an extent that the protein molecules of the digestive enzymes can pass straight into the cancer cell and cause it to dissolve (Wolf).

The blood-borne defence is based mainly on the continued presence, in effective quantity, of specific enzymes and of non-specific protein-digesting enzymes. It seems that the strength of the defences is directly proportional to the quantity of proteases in the blood.

Animal experiments have demonstrated that enzyme therapy can be used to break down cancer cells. In human patients, enzymes attack those cancer cells which are always circulating freely in the blood, and cause them to dissolve. They also digest fibrin clots which may have formed on the walls of blood vessels. It is known that such clots can make it easier for cancer cells to enter into healthy tissue. Enzymes therefore dissolve freely circulating cancer cells and they clean the blood vessels; in this way they help to prevent the development of secondary tumours.

Enzymes also attack tumour tissue. The doses required for this depend on the sensitivity, the size, the rate of growth and the blood supply of the tumour, as well as on other factors. Enzymes also help to prevent the toxic products of the tumour which are circulating in the blood from intoxicating the organism; those normally employed for treatment are nontoxic, even if given in very high doses.

In 1973, when these words were being written, there were many surgeons, radiotherapists and chemotherapists who believed that despite their vast resources—all their knowledge, all their superb equipment, all their ingenious drugs, all their skills and devotions—their best efforts were too often inadequate. Too many children are denied a fair life span, too many adults experience long periods of pain and indignity.

The conventional thinking of today still maintains that the first line of attack should be surgery, unless the malignancy is leukaemia or an allied disease where chemotherapy is called upon. But surgery *takes something away*, it is by its nature mutilatory and is the form of treatment human beings fear most (Farber). The second line of attack is radio-therapy. The "beam" machine cannot be manipulated with the same fine precision as the surgeon's scalpel; it can harm healthy tissue.

Chemotherapy has still to reach the stage where it can achieve more with less side-effects. The promises of hormone and enzyme treatments have yet to be realised; at best they are now no more than additional tools for the surgeon and radiotherapist.

Yet the localistic approach has now dictated the treatment for a hundred years in terms of surgery, seventy years in terms of radiology, thirty years in terms of chemotherapy. After a century of unceasing effort in research, after expending enormous intellectual and material resources, one question above all others needs to be asked: what results have been achieved?

The sobering fact must be faced: only one in every five cancer patients can actually be cured by these methods.

In about sixty out of every hundred cancer cases, the disease is so far advanced by the time it is diagnosed that neither surgery nor radiotherapy can offer prospects of a cure. These patients are given up from the moment of diagnosis as being untreatable, and therefore incurable. They become the "primary incurables".

In about forty cases out of every hundred, surgery and radiation can offer some prospects of success. But, according to all available statistical data, half of these patients, who, after all, have only been treated symptomatically, sooner or later develop local recurrences or secondary tumours. Like the "primary incurables" they are then deemed to be beyond further surgical or radiological intervention, are also pronounced incurable, and left to their fate as hopeless cases. They become the "secondary incurables".

This leaves about twenty out of every hundred who can expect a cure by conventional methods. That has been the situation for many years. The overwhelming majority of cancer patients can expect no help from treatments which are based on the localistic principle only—not now, nor in the future.

It must be clear to everybody—researchers, clinicians and patients—that something must be fundamentally wrong with therapeutic methods used for the past century, if, in spite of ever-intensified research, and almost limitless supplies of money, the problem of cancer has not been solved.

Periodically, the medical journals contain reports that fifty percent of cancers could be cured if only they could be diagnosed early enough; these reports are really a clarion call for the development of improved early diagnostic techniques. But thirty years of practical experience shows too clearly, and sadly, that early screening is not the magic bullet which will produce a higher cure rate. A variety of early diagnostic techniques have been in use since 1940, but the proportion of cures has only marginally increased.

Yet I, too, believe that fifty percent—and more—of all cancer patients can be cured. But, in my opinion, such a decisive improvement can only be achieved when there is a fundamental change in our basic attitude—when the localist approach is abandoned and the whole-body approach to the disease adopted.

4

Early Stages

SYMPTOMATIC TREATMENT CAN BE HARMFUL WHEREVER IN NATURE IT is applied to the soil, plants, animals, human beings—or in medicine. History is filled with examples of sincere men who were swayed too easily by new thoughts and theories and by new developments in technology and chemistry which they used as the bases for clinical practice. Nowhere is this more evident than in the field of cancer, where the organised, implacable methods of healing have become a matter of prejudice rather than the results of enlightened investigation of treatment that is aimed at the long-term support of the patient.

Today, there are doctors, through training and entrenched attitudes, who firmly believe cancer is largely an incurable disease; that any attempt to deviate beyond the medical norm is doomed to failure. They refuse to recognise, or accept, the fundamental idea that a healthy body has the capacity to keep all its billions of cells functioning properly; that a vigorous host can prevent any abnormal growth; that the pre-requisite of any successful cancer therapy is to bring the organism back to that normal physiology *while at the same time* attacking the localised tumour. That is the aim of whole-body therapy.

There is a need to state again some beliefs based on the whole-body concept of cancer which are fundamental to the understanding of the therapy based upon it.

1. Cancer is not a localised illness but a specific generalised, chronic,

48

degenerative disease; before any malignant growth can start, the function of the organism must have been abnormal.

2. Cancer develops when there is a breakdown of the body's resistance against cancer; the body's cells which can develop into cancer cells, exist in every human being. In the reproduction of life they have an essential role to play. Even when these cells behave abnormally, the body's natural defence can combat them. It is when this defence breaks down that the disease begins to flourish.

3. Cancer cells, like normal ones, stay biologically in contact and exchange reaction to the general metabolic processes which are fundamentally all the same for all cells, whether normal or malignant cells. From that statement grows another, and far more important one: tumours are only symptoms of a general disease which are different in their degree and temporary course from other proliferation producing metabolic processes. Tumours should never be regarded as a special type of local disease, but as a late-stage symptom of a generalised illness affecting the whole body. In short, the curing of cancer can best be achieved by not only attacking the localised tumours but also by the restoration of the entire metabolism and the body's natural defence systems.

Before examining this combination treatment in detail, it is essential to understand some basic facts on the whys and wherefores of cancer.

The first is concerned with the origin of cancer cells. Cancer cells resemble the normal cell types from which they came. However, as the malignancy develops, the tumour cells have a tendency to become more "primitive", and to more clearly resemble each other. Observations of the English pathologist L. G. Laijtha confirmed in 1970 that during carcinogenesis many of the cell changes appear to be losses of properties. These observations, however, do not explain the cause for the cell changes. There is a long list of theories that stretch back to the nineteenth century. Many of the early ideas were less concerned with the question of *why* a tumour developed in the body—something that could not then be answered with scientific accuracy—and more concerned with the study of the tumour and the mechanism which caused the cancer cell to originate.

Impetus to this research was provided by Virchow, whose "Irritation Theory" found wide acceptance in 1863 with its claim that malignant neoplasms developed more frequently in organs subject to mechanical or chemical irritation. The theory did not explain one essential question: how and why such irritant factors transformed a normal cell into a cancer cell?

In 1875 Cohnheim produced his theory of embryonic remnants, arguing that embryonic growth which had become quiescent could be reactivated at any time by external stimuli, producing benign or malignant tumours.

Still other theories gained credence. Among them was Otto War-burg's Respiration Theory, which earned him a second Nobel Prize. Warburg argued that if the respiratory enzymes in the mitochondria of the cell are damaged, the cell becomes unable to utilize oxygen. A year after Warburg's work created wide interest, the French biologists, Jacob, Lwoff, and Monod studied the molecular processes leading to mutation. In 1965 they, too, received a Nobel Prize for their Rep-ressor Theory.

Meanwhile another avenue of research continued into pathogenic organisms, prompted by the work of the English surgeon J. Adams who had reported in 1801 that he had seen "worm like parasites" in cells from newly operated breast cancers. Hundreds of scientists have since made it their life-work to look for a specific pathogen causing cancer. In experimental studies, cancer could only be transferred with constant success by injecting whole cancer cells; the injection of pure cultures of bacteria parasitising in cancer cells did not lead to the development of cancer in every case.

Micro-organisms of the bacterial type were therefore unlikely to cause cancer; the assumption grew that an extremely small virus was responsible. Proof was offered by Peyton Rous, the American researcher in 1910. He reported producing experimental tumours by inoculating healthy animals with a cell and bacteria-free filtrate which had been produced from a chicken-sarcoma. Later, in the 1930s Shope and Bittner succeeded in transmitting tumours from mammals by means of a filtrable virus.

Further impetus came in 1957 from W. M. Stanley, the Nobel Prize-winning biologist, who argued that cancer, in animals or man, arose from a single virus-induced biological mechanism which was probably present in every normal cell.

The belief that cancer is caused by micro-organisms has now found world-wide acceptance and a great deal of effort is being expanded by

many investigators in numerous laboratories into isolating one particular strain or another.

One of the more interesting avenues has been pursued by Franz
Gerlach, the Viennese pathologist and microbiologist. He has established
that specific micro-organisms, called Mycoplasma, may be found in
every malignant tumour or cancer cell, and that Mycoplasma plays a
contributive role in the transition from normal to malignant cells.

There are many more scientific theories; they all have one common
factor: they support the argument that cancer is a systemic disease of
the whole organism from the outset and that no cancer cell, whatever
its origin, can produce a malignant tumour unless the organism has
been primed to do so.

Even a casual study of scientific cancer literature only confirms the
idea that the disease must be understood and treated primarily as a
chronic systemic illness of the whole body. Two examples will suffice.
In 1951 H. Druckrey, a German researcher, put forward the hypothesis
that the development and dissemination of cancer becomes possible by
the weakening or loss of the body's natural resistance which destroys
cancer cells that develop constantly and normally in a healthy organism.
Druckrey argued that natural resistance to cancer cells is incapacitated as
a consequence of the complex summation of noxious substances and
damage which has occurred sometimes a long time before to the
organism; these noxious substances lead to a complex chronic metabolic
disturbance and prepare the soil for what I have described as a "tumour
milieu". In 1962 Sir David Smithers, then Cancer Adviser to the
British Government's Department of Health, suggested that cancer is a
disease of organisation and not a disease of cells; its field of study is the
science of organismal organisation; it cannot be encompassed simply
by cytology.

From such theories, coupled with my own intensive clinical experience, it is possible to assess cancer in terms of being a systemic disease.

There is every reason to believe, as Druckrey claimed, that cancer
cells may arise at any time in the body, and that the risk of them doing
so steadily increases with age. Equally, if it were indeed true that every
primary cell which became malignant developed into a tumour, then
everybody would get cancer. That this does not happen confirms the
fact that the body is able to defend itself, using its own natural resources
to withstand, and destroy, the threat of a malignant cell, or cells.

But there comes a point where the defence system can no longer cope because it has been damaged through a variety of causes. The organism then becomes unable to combat cancer cells or prevent them multiplying. That is the moment when the host is able to produce a malignant tumour—and thus develop cancer. At this late stage, crucial factors are combined: a reduction in the natural resistance, and an environment in which a tumour may develop—the "tumour milieu". In combination, they are often deadly, giving little chance for orthodox methods of cancer treatment to succeed.

The most logical way to real success in curing cancer is to explore the underlying early causes of the disease which eventually lead to a tumour.

These early stages are difficult to discern. They are usually hidden, they are not clinically apparent, and they are diverse. However, they provide the foundation on which the entire process and progress of cancer is based.

In 1953, I formalised my concept of the pathogenesis of cancer. It assumes that cancer is a very specific, chronic, general disease of the entire organism whose development I have divided into five phases which are interdependent, often overlap but generally follow consecutively. These phases are:

1. causal factors, leading to
2. secondary damages, leading to
3. tumour milieu and lowered resistance, leading to
4. ability to form tumours and the resulting tumour formation, leading to
5. tumour symptoms.

During phases 1 to 4, the chronic, general disease of the whole organism develops. In referring to the cancer disease I therefore mean the sum total of all the phases in the causal chain, and not just the late stage symptom, the tumour.

My working hypothesis, describing the five phases, is shown in simplified, schematic, form on the facing page.

Pre- and post-natal endogenous and exogenous causal factors (I), by mutative, toxic, neural, or sensitising effects via the transit mesenchyme, can produce secondary damage (II) in cells, in the control mechanisms (nervous and hormonic systems), in the detoxifying, excretory, and defence systems.

Figure 1. Hypothesis of Pathogenesis of Cancer

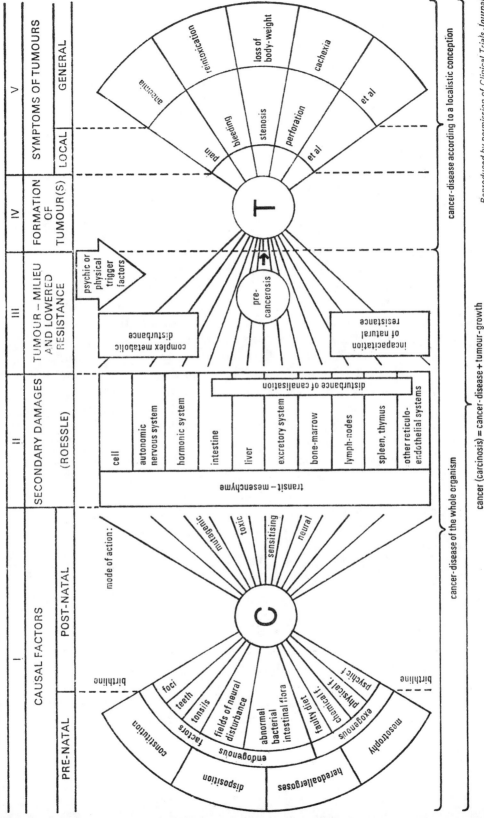

In particular, affects on excretory canalisation may lead to complex metabolic disturbances which lower natural resistance and produce an imbalanced situation gradually developing into a tumour milieu (III).

From such primary, precancerous conditions, a secondary precancerous condition may develop at a site of least resistance, and when the defence potency is lowered further, an oncogenous condition may result in malignant growth (IV and V).

In phase one, first we must look at the prenatal factors. From the moment of conception until death, the human organism is exposed to a wide variety of influences which may be either beneficial or damaging; the thalidomide tragedy has shown the disastrous consequences of such prenatal influences. Anything which is harmful to the expectant mother—environmental pollution, drugs, nicotine, the wrong diet, mental stress, alcohol and other stimulants—will affect the organism of the foetus. The child may be much more seriously affected than the mother, not only from chemical agents, but also from infectious conditions such as German measles and other virus diseases, or from the effects of radiation. Nor is the influence of harmful environmental factors limited to one generation. There is an abundance of evidence to show that this damage can be handed down from one generation to another; in such circumstances the new-born child comes into the world with a mortgage which is the sum total of all damage sustained in previous generations and imprinted in the genetic structures. There is no doubt that this negative dowry is partly responsible for subsequent deterioration in health and the increase in chronic illness. This can be clearly seen in the constitution of new generations of babies whose mothers and fathers and grand-parents before them have been exposed, and expose themselves, to the perils of our modern life-style.

Constitution is a term describing the disposition, the individual characteristics of a person which have been conditioned through hereditary and environmental factors. These manifest themselves in a person's physical build, individual fitness, reactions, adaptability, resilience and, of course, his susceptibility to disease.

Although a constitution predisposed by hereditary factors towards illness will always mean the entire organism is endangered, it is very often only one particular organ which becomes afflicted. This weak spot is "the site of least resistance", where chronic irritation may initially make itself most strongly felt, and where chronic diseases, such as cancer, will become manifest. Here, too, hereditary traits play a part, acting as the focal point for an illness. I have found that these focal points (the local disposition) can be traced back through a family's generations: a grandfather had a weak stomach; his son had an ulcer; the grandson had stomach cancer.

Such observations show there are deep-rooted causes for all chronic diseases, and that a cure cannot be achieved by merely treating the prevailing symptoms and ignoring the predisposing congenital dowry such as the inherited residual toxicoses which are present in every cell of the organism and result from infections suffered from earlier generations. These are called heredo-allergoses.

Carl Spengler, assistant medical director and protégé of the German bacteriologist and tuberculosis specialist, Robert Koch, has defined inherited residual toxicoses of major importance as "masked" tuberculosis and "masked" syphilis. From his considerable clinical experience Spengler concluded that residuals of active or latent tuberculosis in man may lead to a sensitisation of the body cells which he defined as "masked". They often produce chronic illnesses, and also those conditions that prepare the way for cancer. Spengler argued it was not enough to treat symptomatically, but causally.

In the course of his investigations, Spengler demonstrated that there are four types of pathogen for tuberculosis, and two of these produce the disease in humans.

In the organism, the specific foreign protein of inherited tuberculosis, tubercle protein, produces a sensitisation which may in turn evoke many different symptoms and signs. These constitute the syndrome of "masked" tuberculosis. According to Spengler all human beings are born to a varying extent with inherited residual tuberculosis, and this therefore provides a permanent contributory cause in chronic disease— and must always be taken into account and treated. In the course of time, sensitisation of the organism through this inherited toxic state may result in the gradual, insidious development of functional disorders in organs and organic systems. This toxic effect continues throughout life and is one of the key factors in the development of chronic disease.

Spengler also showed that all known pathogens are subject to pleomorphic cycling, changing from primitive phases as small as a virus to bacterial or fungal stages. The organism causing syphilis may also be found in the cells of the human organism in "virus small" form—even if infection with syphilis never occurred in a person's lifetime.

It must be assumed that the universal presence of inherited syphilis is a memento of the sixteenth century. At that time the disease was brought to Europe from America and spread like wildfire through the population. Those who did not die from it were left with a "residual toxicosis", which has been passed down through the generations and often given new impetus through reinfection.

This "masked" syphilis is far more prevalent today than is generally recognised; it also seems to be a contributory cause to diseases with proliferative features and morbid growth. The syphilis pathogen is known to have an affinity to the nervous and skeletal systems and to the skin, and so these organic systems are especially sensitised by the proteinic toxins of masked syphilis.

Physicians who believe in treating the organism as a whole accept that the tendency to react to toxic stimulus with proliferation rather than inflammation—as seen in cancer patients—may be caused, or enhanced by these inherited toxic states. Medically qualified homoeo-paths and naturopaths, trained to observe various constitutional aspects, have always looked upon the inherited toxic states, particularly tuber-culosis and syphilis, as the pace-makers of cancer.

There is also a third one, endobiosis. Endobiotic organisms are microbes living in symbiosis with the healthy host organisms. Under certain conditions, these organisms change into a pathogenic form, which can have a major role in the genesis of chronic disease, including cancer.

Masked tuberculosis, masked syphilis, and parasitic endobiosis form corner stones in the development of chronic disease, and can be regarded as the indirect causes of cancer. These causal factors produce the morbidly changed soil on which more recent genetic factors, for instance residual toxicosis of later infections can develop and produce chronic organic illness.

The next prenatal causal factor to be considered is mesotrophy (Kollath), the slow, often barely perceptible deterioration in health caused by deficient nutrition which has persisted over several genera-tions. By deficient nutrition I mean a diet usually rich in calories, but poor in vitamins and minerals. We shall be looking at this situation in more detail in chapter nine.

To sum up: the four prenatal factors—constitution, disposition (innate organic weaknesses), inherited residual toxicoses (heredo-allergoses), mesotrophy—represent a latent potential for disease which everyone inherits from his forebears. As we have seen, every human being is mortgaged at birth; today, healthy new-born babies are practically unknown. Statistics show the mortgage is getting bigger with each generation. It seems people show an increasing disposition to develop chronic disease in direct relation to exposure to the exogenous influences of modern civilisation. This is the only possible explanation why cancer has increased numerically, and why even children are increasingly afflicted. The onset of the disease comes earlier.

In the course of life, postnatal causal factors are added to the existing prenatal factors, and these represent more obvious, and more immediate, causes for the development of disease.

Now let us turn to the endogenous postnatal causal factors.

1. Head foci—in teeth, tonsils, sinuses etc.

For forty years it has been generally accepted that chronic infections in the teeth and tonsils may cause damage to the organism. They can produce malfunction of the natural defences, and are so important in cancer and other chronic diseases that their role will be discussed in detail in chapter seven.

2. Disturbance fields.

The distant effects of a "focus" may arise through toxic, allergic, or neural mechanisms. A centre of irritation causing distant symptoms by the neural route is called a field of disturbance. Chronic diseases are partly caused by foci of disturbance. Their contribution to disease can only be eliminated by expert diagnosis and treatment of every focus.

3. Abnormal intestinal flora.

Shortly after birth, physiological microbes begin to grow on all mucous membranes in the infant's organism. These colonies are of great importance to the health and life expectancy of Man; one sign of a sound constitution is a healthy intestinal flora. It has also been shown that disease is frequently preceded by abnormalities in flora. Thus, health and bacteria are interdependent. Further, a causal relation between abnormal flora and cancer has been definitely established.

There are also exogenous postnatal causal factors.

5. Faulty diet.

First and foremost among "external" causes which undermine health is faulty nutrition concomitant with modern civilisation. The consequences of this can be passed down through generations as already mentioned.

6. Chemical factors from the environment.

Many chemical compounds will, under certain conditions, induce chronic illness, and become a direct cause in the development of cancer. There are, for instance, the occupational forms of cancer caused by coal-tar, aniline, arsenic, and cancer caused by smoking.

Foreign substances which we take up daily, and involuntarily, with our food, water, and the air we breathe, may have effects on health. These substances include the colouring, flavouring, and preservative agents in food, the insecticides sprayed on fruit and vegetables, pesticides, petrol fumes, industrial smog, and last, but not least, the many drugs our civilisation dispenses.

Toxins which have entered the organism must be converted to compounds which do not react and can be eliminated. In the course of time the detoxicating and eliminatory capacities of the liver, intestine, and kidneys are no longer adequate, and as we shall see, this aggravates the secondary damage caused by these toxins in the organism.

All exogenous toxins are anti-enzymatic agents and may contribute to the development of neoplastic disease in two ways: firstly, by causing First Cancer Cells to arise in the "weak points" of the organism; secondly, because the secondary damage they have caused will later give rise to a tumour milieu and depress natural resistance. Without the tumour milieu and depressed resistance, First Cancer Cells cannot multiply and lead to tumour growth.

7. Physical factors from the environment.

Physical irritants may also cause chronic diseases, including cancer. For instance, sailors subject to sunburn over many years sometimes develop skin cancer; scars from burns and irradiation are weak points and therefore "sites of preference" for the development of carcinoma.

Prolonged exposure to X-rays and radio-active emissions can cause not only a local area to be disposed to cancer, but also cause secondary damage to internal organs, and above all, a marked and persisting loss of resistance. As the result of the nuclear tests, and the use of high-energy material in atomic power stations, radio-active fall-out has contaminated the surface of the earth. Traces of carcinogenic elements are now present in all our food and drink. Although the levels of radio-activity at present are not high enough to be considered a cancer risk in themselves, their accumulative effect certainly aggravates that of innumerable other carcinogenic factors which surround us.

8. Psychic stress.

Many elements in the environment may not be specifically pathogenic but still contribute indirectly to the development or manifestation of serious illness. These include anything liable to cause psychic stress. Such situations can reduce vitality, gradually break down natural resistance, and finally show themselves in physical illness. The wrong job, frequent trouble with superiors, with colleagues, with the marriage partner—these are just a few of the more common stress situations which may contribute materially to the secondary damages which in turn may lead to a tumour milieu and further lowering of resistance.

Newton, Friedmann and Rasmussen have shown that animals given loving care, survived much longer than those kept in isolation and never fondled. Man, too, thrives in a stress-reduced, harmonious environment. A tumour may be triggered by a stress situation.

Many researchers have described a characteristic psychic pattern seen in cancer patients: they tend to suppress inner problems, keeping a tight control on their feelings; they are afraid of personal relationships with emotional involvement, and shrink back to a defensive position when faced with the possibility of making deeper contact at the level of the soul and spirit.

Other workers have stated that cancer patients have often had a joyless childhood. Those who grow up without a warm family atmosphere, who are deprived of mother love or parental care during childhood, will often find themselves unable to form and create significant, close, human relationships later in life; they may also find it impossible to give true expression to their love and try to suppress their emotions. According to Kissen (Glasgow), and others, this may contribute to a cancer disposition.

Although by necessity somewhat simplified, the foregoing has been an attempt to show something of the many different causal factors, effective before and after birth, which can indirectly contribute to the development of cancer. From this it can be argued the disease cannot be ascribable to a single cause, but to a number of factors. It is clear that our knowledge is inadequate: we can never know to what extent individual factors have contributed to the development of a malignancy; they affect various mechanisms in varying degrees; many have multiple action; they may reinforce or potentiate one another.

The first and most urgent step in the whole-body approach to cancer is to trace these causes, and to thoroughly eliminate them. The more successfully we remove the causal factors, the greater is the chance that we will have stopped secondary damage which would have been produced by them.

The causal factors mentioned may take effect by various mechanisms: mutation, toxic effects, sensitisation, neural effects. But what they all have in common is the ability to produce secondary damages in cells, organs, and organic systems.

My own clinical experience has shown that it is essential to approach an illness, especially a chronic one like cancer, from the basis that the damaged organ is only a symptom of a number of deeper factors. There is, for instance, clear evidence that the effect of poisons or toxins on the body over many years, often over a lifetime, causes severe damage. This kind of damage has been defined by those two excellent exponents of causal treatment, Grote and Roessle.

It is known that causal factors take effect via the transit mesenchyme: damage to cells of the respective organs comes about by this route. I shall deal firstly with the transit mesenchyme and the cell, and then later with secondary damage to organs.

Life in the cell, the maintenance and activity of its functional structures, depends on the presence of certain substrates and energy providers. These must be constantly available to the cell from its environment. Having to take up nutrient substances and give off unwanted products, the cell must rely on a steady exchange of substances with its environment, known as the "flow equilibrium" (Schade).

Three independent systems link cells to each other and to the organism as a whole. They are the nervous system, the blood, and the lymph vessels. These systems remain separated from the cells by a space, known as the transit distance; the to-and-fro exchange between the cells and the transport systems must proceed across this space. The cells are therefore completely surrounded by a service area of soft connective tissues. Causal factors reaching the organs via the blood will first of all act on the soft connective tissues.

Soft connective tissue is the term used for the unstructured mesenchymal tissue which links the formed elements of the body (W. E. Ehrich). The frame structure of connective tissue consists of a network or reticulum of cells. These cells can be divided into groups with different functions:

Large reticulum cells—these develop into monocytes and become the end-cells (peripheral synapses) of sympathetic nerves.
Small reticulum cells—these become lymphocytes (immunocytes) and form the end-organs of parasympathetic nerves.
Intercalary reticulum cells ("bright cells")—these are neurohumoral cells and produce serotonin.

Connective tissue has a multiplicity of functions. It is responsible for all metabolic exchanges between blood and parenchyma cells and for this reason has also been called the "colloidal river bed of fluids". Because of its mediating or "transit" function, the soft connective tissue is nowadays generally called the "transit mesenchyme" to distinguish it from certain specific forms of mesenchyme.

Connective tissue maintains a constant metabolic exchange and therefore osmotic pressure, an optimal electrolyte balance, and the acid-base equilibrium. Because of its ability to maintain isotonicity in the body fluids by storing protein, salts and water, the connective tissue has also been called the pre-kidney. Foreign proteins such as micro-organisms or products of degradation within the body, for instance from disease foci, are swallowed up in the process of phagocytosis and digested by connective tissue cells. Foreign substances and environmental toxins reaching the "smallest tissue element" via the blood stream are captured and chemically bound in connective tissue. Carcinogenic toxins from the environment may be bound by the positive valency bonds of mesenchymal ground substance. Connective tissue therefore also has a clearing and storage function.

The functional capacity of the connective tissue cell—and of any other cell—is primarily determined by the state of the cellular systems of information and respiration. It is these systems which suffer secondary damage first and foremost by the earlier causal factors. As a result, the organ-specific activity of the mesenchymal cell is reduced. It has been known for a long time that deficiencies in vitamins, bio-elements, oxygen and other vital substances may be detrimental to the mesenchymal cell. Clinical experience and the results of experimental studies have also shown that the mesenchyme may be damaged by toxins, that in the mesenchymal cell cancerogenic toxins produce damage which is visible under the microscope, in the form of "turbid swelling".

The functions of the nervous system and the mesenchyme are interdependent, and disruption in one system will also affect the other, leading among other things to allergic reactions.

When the mesenchyme is no longer able to take out of circulation surplus acids, bases, and other metabolites affecting the organism, the regulatory function of connective tissue is impaired and the composition of the blood becomes abnormal.

The functions of the mesenchyme may become exhausted because the volume of substances to be stored is greater than the storage capacity. If this happens, the mesenchyme will become "blocked", with, as we shall soon see, most serious consequences.

The most common causes producing secondary damage to the cells are:

Virus infections, including inherited infections.

Deficiencies in vitamins, bio-elements, oxygen and other essential substances.

Chemical toxins which reach the cell from dental and tonsillar foci, from the intestine and from other sites, or are taken in with the food or the air.

Physical influences from the environment, which may either cause mutation, or simply change the electrical properties of genes affecting their charge or ability to oscillate.

Numerous experimental studies have shown that mitochondrial structures and functions suffer damage from many different toxins, and also from deficiency in oxygen or essential factors.

Damage or destruction of mitochondrial structures will of course always involve all the biochemical processes localised within them. Aerobic respiration is inhibited. The loss of mitochondrial function causes an "enzyme defect". Many biochemical processes will then be incomplete or faulty.

Damaged mitochrondria can recover if the factors responsible for the damage are completely eliminated.

The structural and functional defects giving rise to complex functional disorder in cells may be summarised as follows:

Variable degrees of enzyme defect in the organelles, particularly in the aerobic structures of the cell and those containing DNA and RNA.
Reduction or loss of aerobic biochemical function.
Changes in membrane potentials, in extreme cases depolarisation.
Cellular acidosis.
Changes in cellular proteins.
Reduction or total loss of organ-specific functional capacity of the cell.
Altered response to neurohumoral stimulus.

The nervous and glandular organs concerned with regulation of the vital processes are called the vegetative system. The nerve elements are designated the autonomic nervous system; the glandular control organs are known as the incretory glands, or "endocrinium".

The autonomic nervous system comprises two partial systems with opposite functions: the sympathetic system which directs the use of energy, and the parasympathetic which is responsible for the availability of reserves.

Autonomic stimuli may reach the organs by the hormonal as well as by the neural routes. Hormones, reaching the cell via the blood, may also initiate biochemical processes. As with the nervous system, distinction is made between central and peripheral organs of hormonic regulation.

The diencephalon contains a number of autonomic nerve centres of vital importance and also the centre of hormonal regulation for the organism. The neural parts of the diencephalon are known as the thalamus and the hypothalamus, the glandular parts as the hypophysis (pituitary body) and epiphysis cerebri (pineal body or gland). The thalamus, hypothalamus, pituitary and pineal body are known as the diencephalo-hypophyseal system. The neural and hormonal functions arising from this cannot be separated on any anatomical or functional basis, as they are closely interwoven. The hypophysis produces substances which stimulate the endocrine glands of the periphery to release hormones with specific actions on the organism as a whole.

The thyroid gland is stimulated by the thyrotrophic hormone from the anterior lobe of the hypophysis to produce thyroid hormones. These activate the mitochondria and therefore aerobic metabolism in the cell. Inhibition of thyroid activity will accordingly cause an inhibition of aerobic respiration in the cell, and this will favour the development of cancer.

The parathyroid glands, epithelial bodies, are stimulated by the parathyrotropic hormone of the anterior lobe of the hypophysis to produce substances called parathormone or Collip hormone. These are responsible for calcium, magnesium and phosphate metabolism, and for all enzymatic functions involving calcium, magnesium and phosphates, as co-enzymes, or in any other way.

In the "islet cells" of the pancreas, insulin is produced under the influence of the pancreotropic hormone from the anterior lobe of the hypophysis. Insulin enables the organism to take the carbohydrates ingested with the food and store them in the form of starch. If insufficient insulin is produced, sugar contained in the food we eat remains in solution in the blood and has to be excreted in the urine, a condition known as diabetes.

Several hormones of the anterior lobe of the hypophysis appear to act on the adrenal cortex. Adreno-corticotropic hormones cause the cortex to release glucocorticoids such as cortisone, while the somatotropic hormone of the anterior lobe plays a role in the production of mineralocorticoids, such as desoxycorticosterone. Cortical hormones are essential for oxidative phosphorylation and hence the recovery of energy and aerobic processes within the mitochondria. Inadequate function of the adrenal cortex must therefore result in serious disruption of cellular metabolism.

The genital glands, ovary and testes, are stimulated by the gonadotropic hormones of the anterior lobe of the hypophysis and adrenal to produce sex-specific catalysts which play a role not only for the reproductive organs, but also the organism as a whole.

Neither the neural nor the humoral part of the vegetative system is able on its own to provide for optimal function of the vital processes. Each of the two systems needs collaboration from the other if it is to develop its potential to the full.

F. Hoff described the vegetative system as a chain of functional cycles inseparably linked through the feedback mechanism—like a system of cog wheels. If one of these "cog wheels" moves, all the others in the system would of necessity also have to start moving. Any impulse from one of the functional cycles therefore sets in motion a general vegetative shift. If on the other hand one of the "cog wheels" becomes fixed, unable to move, all the other "wheels" also come to a standstill. In that case, the system cannot adapt easily to any new situation; adaptability gives way to a regulatory freeze. In cancer patients, this tends to be a parasympathicotonic freeze.

The full import of the close relationship between the functional capacity of the vegetative system and the disposition towards disease may be seen if we consider the biology of the nervous system. The smallest functional unit in this system, the neurone, consists of the actual nerve, or ganglion cell, and the nerve fibres connecting the ganglion cell with its terminal organ; this makes up the three-chamber system of the smallest tissue unit.

If the nerve fibre is irritated at any point, this will produce four results:

1. The peripheral part of the nerve fibre loses its ability to receive and conduct stimulus, and degenerates.
2. The nerve fibre is only recharged with energy, and nourished, as long as it is fully connected with its ganglion cell.
3. Nerve fibre and reacting organ therefore perish together.
4. The ganglion cell, condemned to permanent inactivity with the loss of its nerve fibre, gradually also loses the ability to respond to stimulus and dies. Every ganglion cell functions in conjunction with other ganglion cells, and the death of one ganglion cell starts a chain reaction which sooner or later may affect the vegetative system as a whole.

This is known as "neural dystrophy". A local circumscribed neural defect is transmitted by neural pathways and inhibits regeneration within the whole sphere of the nervous system, and accordingly within the whole sphere of the mesenchyme. Local, circumscribed dystrophy may give rise to a complex disturbance of regulatory function and a general dystrophy of neural genesis. This may start from any point in the organism—for instance from a dental or intervertebral disc lesion.

Organs of the vegetative system may be damaged as follows:

They may be directly affected through faulty nutrition, through toxic factors, and through any of the causal factors which produce pathological changes in the organelles and in the biochemical processes of the cell. Indirect damage is transmitted by neural pathways, with any trauma in the periphery inevitably affecting also the transmission system in the organism.

In the development of dystrophy it is immaterial whether the neural damage was due to deficiency in essential factors, to intoxication, to infection, to injury or any other pathogenic factor.

The living organism differs from its non-living environment in its ability to counter pathogenic processes out of its own resources. This is what "life" means: the laws governing the organism are under the overall control of the laws of nature. If the organism's power to control is reduced, this results in illness, and if it is lost altogether this means death (F. Hoff). The regulatory organs, the vegetative system, are therefore responsible for the maintenance of life, and without their help the organism is unable to cope with environmental influences.

Any damage to the vegetative system brings with it loss of vitality, the signs of which are vegetative dystonia and a disposition towards chronic diseases of all kinds. The balanced interplay between sympathicotonic and parasympathicotonic impulses becomes more or less restricted, and sometimes even completely abnormal, resulting in a vegetative "freeze"; the sympathicotonic form of this seems to be characteristic for sarcomas and systemic neoplasia, the parasympathicotonic form for carcinomas.

If the vegetative system is no longer able to make the physical and chemical processes in the organism conform to the laws of the organism, the specific ordering principle concomitant with normal health is absent, and eucrasia, the constant equilibrium of the body fluids, is also lost.

The destructive effects of the causal factors on the vegetative system evolve at many levels, and may be summarised as:

Dystonia of the vegetative system.
Dystrophy of the organism as a whole.
Dyscrasia of the body fluids.

Now let us turn to secondary damage of the intestinal environment.

The human gut may be said to consist of two "fermenting chambers" —the small and the large intestine. These differ anatomically, functionally, and also in their bacterial flora.

The small intestine is the organ for enzymatic digestion where all the digestive juices of the body come together. It is closed off at both ends by ring muscle valves, and is a tube of mucous membrane five metres in length. Every square centimetre of mucosa in the small intestine is covered with three thousand villi, so that its absorbing area is increased to approximately forty square metres, up to fifty times the surface area of the intestinal wall. As a result, foods broken down by enzymatic action are rapidly absorbed. Between eighty and ninety percent of the digested food so absorbed is passed on to the blood.

The digestive capacity of the organ depends on three factors: the food must be "predigested" in the stomach before it is received by the intestine, digestive enzymes must be present in adequate amounts, and the food must remain in the small intestine for a sufficiently long period.

Optimal utilization of food is possible only if it passes from the stomach to the small intestine in small amounts. This will happen if the stomach's contents are sufficiently acidic; if they contain too little or no acid—as is the case when there is cancer of the stomach—then the food enters the small intestine abruptly, and is equally abruptly passed on to the large intestine, there causing internal diarrhoea.

The mucous membrane of the large intestine does not have villi like the small intestine, nor glands producing enzymes. Within hours of birth, its walls are thickly carpeted with colibacilli. Under normal conditions, this carpet makes it impossible for any other organisms, and particularly any that do not belong in the intestine, to get anywhere near the mucosa.

Digestion as such does not take place in the large intestine. The digestive processes which do occur come about as a result of the enzymes added to the food in the stomach and the small intestine. The main function of the large intestine is to withdraw water from its contents and, as we shall see, to eliminate toxins.

As food passes through the intestine, it is not merely broken down into units small enough to be absorbed but it is also in part converted into highly toxic biogenic amines and other ptomaines. Although very toxic, they do not normally endanger the organism because detoxicating systems serve to make toxic substances harmless before they reach the blood stream. The first of the detoxicating systems is the mucous membrane of the intestine. The second is the liver which is called into action if the intestinal system is unable to cope with all the toxins present. Naturally, damage to the intestinal cell reduces its power of detoxication. If this happens, large quantities of toxins will then continue to pass to the liver, and when the capacity of this organ begins to fail, to the systemic circulation. In this case, the body is literally poisoning itself with its own intestinal toxins.

The liver is the biggest gland in the body. Its function is to convert the substances produced after digestion into proteins, carbohydrates, fats, and other substrates and energy-carriers, and to store them in this form. As I have said, the liver is also the second-line detoxicating system, between the intestine and the organism as a whole. All toxins produced in the intermediary metabolism at cellular level, or those coming in from the intestine, are generally converted to nontoxic substances which the body can eliminate. Detoxicated poisons and any unwanted metabolic products are then eliminated with the bile.

Further, the liver also has regulatory functions. It constantly monitors all intermediary metabolic processes, and finally, it produces a considerable quantity of defence enzymes and gamma globulins.

Liver cells are very rich in mitochondria—a quarter of their content may be made up of this small organelle found within the cytoplasm of cells. Because of this, the liver cell is highly susceptible to anything which might damage its mitochondria. Toxic and neural impairment, as well as stress, result in a loss of mitochondrial enzymes. In addition, many constituents of the mitochondria are essential factors which the organism is unable to produce itself and which must be taken in with the food. Any nutritional deficiency will therefore reduce the number and activity of mitochondria.

The detoxicating function of the liver cell is proportionate to the aerobic activity developed by its mitochondria. As long as these organelles are intact and supplied with all necessary vital substances, mitochondria are able to convert even highly dangerous carcinogens into harmless products.

A liver cell subject to continuous vitamin deficiency is unable to counter effectively the daily onslaught of environmental toxins; on the contrary, it will itself sustain damage from those toxins. If the toxic invasion is such that the detoxication systems cannot keep up, the toxins entering the body or those produced within it must then be stored in the cells of the liver, the mesenchyme, and other organs.

To return to the intestine; its purpose is not only—as is generally assumed—to detoxicate and to remove undigested material. Of equal importance is its function as an outlet for toxins produced in the body.

One finds, in all parts of the gastrointestinal tract, glandular cells which excrete such toxin. A considerable volume of the faeces consists of toxic excretions of the intestinal mucosa and of shed mucosal cells. Excretion of toxic material tends to be most active during the night and when fasting.

Even if no food is eaten at all, more than twenty grammes of faeces are evacuated each day. Very active elimination of toxins may sometimes give rise to what the physicians of old called "black bile".

According to Buerger, ulceration of the large intestine seen in cases of uraemia or poisoning by heavy metal suggests the large intestine excretes toxins more actively than any other section of the digestive tract. Indeed, if mercury enters the body—by being inadvertently eaten, or inhaled as a dust or vapour, or even by being absorbed through the skin—the major part of it will be excreted by the intestinal mucosa; however, the most intensive excretion is known to be through the mucosa of the large intestine whose potency with regard to mercury is two to three times that of the rest of the bowels.

The rectum, the lower part of the large intestine, is surrounded by a dense, spongy network of haemorrhoidal veins. If they become enlarged, piles may develop, a situation found particularly when the detoxicating capacity of the liver is overstrained. Physicians of old used blood letting by leeches on those veins, to relieve the liver and the body.

As I have said, I believe the main organ responsible for evacuating the toxic protein is the mucosa of the large intestine—which I call the "filter". For each of my patients I have one hope—to open this "filter". If it becomes blocked, the toxins which should pass into the large intestine cannot enter it, and are retained in the body.

No one can easily explain how the "filter" becomes blocked; there is no way of proving it by clinical examination of a living patient, and autopsy also proves nothing. But, in my experience, by examining the tongue we can assess the excretory activity of the mucous membranes in the digestive tract, and also determine whether the filter system has been blocked—the tongue accurately mirrors the state of the intestines.

A normal tongue is always wet and mucous; with chronic diseases, including cancer, it is often dry and has little or no coating of mucus—signifying that the excretory functions have been impaired and that most likely the "filter" has been blocked, During treatment, the tongue will become coated and its colour will change, becoming white, grey, steel-blue, or even black; the thicker the coating and the darker it becomes, the more intensive is the activity of the excretory system in ridding the body of toxins. But if the situation is not corrected, if the "filter" remains blocked, the poisonous toxins build up in the mesenchyme, and are eventually forced into the stomach, causing violent spells of vomiting; into the small intestine, causing internal diarrhoea; and into the subcutaneous tissue, causing sweating which continues for weeks and the typical yellow colouring of cancer patients.

If the body is unable to rid itself of such toxins, the result, eventually, is death. That is why I place so much emphasis on "opening the filter", by, among other methods, employing fever treatment and attending to the head foci, as we shall see in later chapters.

As I have indicated, the skin is not just a protective and sensory organ, but is also a major metabolic and eliminatory system. Even if one is not involved in physical exertion of any kind, the body gives off between five hundred and nine hundred grammes of sweat per day, containing between ten and eighteen grammes of solids. Thus the skin has been quite rightly described as the third kidney.

Man's skin contains more sweat glands than woman's; secretory activity in the skin is greater in men than in women, and also more important since women are able to eliminate part of their endogenous toxins with the menses. If elimination via the skin is reduced, this therefore tends to have a particularly bad effect on the male. As for women, it has long been known that those with a strong, regular, menstrual period are less likely to develop cancer than those whose menses is weak or irregular, or has stopped altogether.

Obviously, the urinary organs have an important eliminatory function. The kidneys filter out unwanted metabolic products and toxins, maintaining a constant concentration of all normal constituents in the blood. Normally, the volume of urine excreted depends on the degree of protein metabolism and the water intake, and also to some extent on the performance of the other eliminatory organs. Low fluid intake, perspiration, diarrhoea, and a diet low in protein will reduce urinary volume. Taking plenty of fluids and a diet rich in protein will increase it.

Urinary elimination is concerned mainly with the end products of protein metabolism. A large proportion of nitrogen is synthetised in the liver and transported to the kidneys by the blood. All foreign substances circulating in the blood and all other toxins—including the highly toxic polysaccharides from tumours—are eliminated by the parenchyma of the kidney. If renal function is impaired, the concentration of urinary solids in the blood and tissues rises. The body will then try to eliminate unwanted material by other routes, so that there may be vomiting, diarrhoea, or increased sweating. A total renal failure cannot be compensated by the other eliminatory systems of the body.

What are the consequences of damage to the eliminatory functions? If these systems have been damaged and are no longer able to eliminate "homotoxins" completely, the organism will try to live with those toxins that persist and, as far as possible, to deposit them in the connective tissues. Reckeweg (1955), who has comprehensively studied the condition, has rather aptly called this the "storage phase". If the volume of unwanted material is greater than the capacity for detoxication, storage capacity will finally be exhausted, and the toxins may then pass into the blood and tissues. Obesity, arteriosclerosis, varicose veins, the formation of calculi, dropsy, the development of cysts and rheumatic nodules are examples of the results of this depositing stage, the beginning of what may become a deadly chain reaction.

When the deposits of homotoxins have caused pathological changes in the cellular structures, the storage phase becomes one of impregnation, resulting, for example, in toxic damage to the liver and kidneys, chronic inflammation of nerves, benign lymphoma, and elephantiasis.

Once toxic impregnation has led to degenerative destruction of the cells concerned, the kidney or liver may contract, there may be paralysis and arthritis, atrophy of the bone marrow, and other serious conditions.

Any tissue that has sustained particularly severe damage may finally become malignant. The degenerative phase has thus turned into one of deviation or neoplasia, and tumour formation then occurs (Reckeweg).

Chronic damage to the eliminatory mechanism will therefore always have immensly serious consequences for the organism.

The body's third line of resistance to disease is that of the reticulo-endothelial system—the RES—which consists of certain cells and tissues of mesenchymal origin scattered throughout all parts of the body, often in conjunction with the transit mesenchyme, and also forming specific organs. Tissues of this type are found in the red and white bone marrow, the spleen, thymus, lymph nodes, pleura and peritoneum, meninges and vascular endothelium. Together, these tissues make up the defence system of the body.

Like all connective tissue cells, those of the RES are able to separate from the reticulae tissue, where they are linked with other cells, and change into wandering cells, entering diseased organs and there taking up the battle with pathogenic organisms or cancer cells. Their defence activity is based on specific and non-specific substances produced by the cells of the mesenchyme.

The specific substances are proteases; these develop proteolytic activity only in relation to anything which is not, or no longer, a normal constituent of the organism—they do not dissolve intact healthy cells. Protective enzymes of this type are the bacteriolysins, the cytolysins (in diseased organs, these dissolve cells which are no longer viable), and the carcinolysins (enzymes which dissolve cancer cells). Abderhalden's test may be used to demonstrate the presence of any of these enzymes in the urine.

Protective enzymes are only produced when needed. Thus carcinolysins will only be present if cancer cells have developed in the body or if they have been injected to give active immunisation. However, a healthy organism is able to resist cancer cells, or carcinogens, even without protective enzymes, because the blood always contains a number of "non-specific" protective factors against all potential pathogens.

Ginsberg and Horsfall gave the first description of virus-inactivating serum factors. The best known of these is properdin, a mixture of alpha-, beta-, and gamma-globulins. According to Southam, it only becomes active in the presence of activating polysaccharides, magnesium ions, and other activators. If a tumour is present, properdin is effective solely against necrotic tumour cells (Isliker).

Mast cells (basophilic granulocytes) and lymphocytes (immunocytes) as well as other connective tissue cells contain heparinoids able to dissolve cancer cells.

The non-specific digestive enzymes in the blood also have a protective function. They too are able to dissolve cancer cells if they are produced in sufficient quantity, and not inactivated too rapidly by antienzymes.

As with any other cell, the structure and functional capacity of RES cells are damaged by deficiency states and by toxins, and the mesenchymal protective substances are then no longer produced in sufficient quantity and quality; phagocytic activity against cancer cells and diseased organic cells is diminished, and the detoxicating power of the RES cells reduced; secondary damage has occurred.

For a long time, localists thought it was wishful thinking that the body possessed natural resistance to cancer. However, spontaneous regression of tumours the size of a fist, or even a head, has been definitely confirmed in both humans and animals. According to Domagk, such regression shows there must be substances in the organism capable of destroying cancer cells, and these substances must be produced by the organism itself.

Many researchers have observed the processes which occur in connective tissues if there is malignant growth. It has been reported, for instance, that with spontaneous regression of mouse tumours, the reactive tissue consisted in the main of lymphocytes and plasma cells. Similar observations have been made by Fischer, Herzog, Hueck, Fromme, Fischer-Wasels, and others. Culture experiments may also be used to demonstrate the anti-cancer activity of the reticulo-endothelial systems—the RES. I have found this activity confirmed again and again in my own clinical experience.

But the damage caused by toxins entering the body goes beyond the organs they first come in contact with. As with all other cells, the structure and functional capacity of RES cells are damaged, and mesenchymal protective substances are then no longer produced in sufficient quantity and quality.

Phagocytic activity against cancer cells and diseased organic cells is also diminished, and the detoxicating power of the RES cells reduced.

The mesenchymal organs may suffer secondary damage as well. One of these is the red marrow. Its function is to produce red blood corpuscles. If the bone marrow cells are damaged, the number and quality of red corpuscles is reduced. This deficiency leads to anaemia and reduction in the oxygen-transport capacity of the blood. And this in turn means that not enough oxygen is made available to the tissues.

The body's "drainage" system can be very seriously affected by secondary damage. Drainage is a descriptive term customarily used for the biological processes concerned with the neutralisation and elimination of toxins and waste products. It therefore includes two components: the detoxicating function of the intestinal mucosa, the intestinal flora, the liver, the RES and the ground tissue; and the eliminatory functions of the intestine, the liver, the skin, the kidneys, the uterus, and other excretory epithelial tissue.

The function of the drainage system is to keep body fluids and tissues clear, and to render harmless and remove any toxins and substances not required for physiological processes.

Causal factors can lead to secondary damage in the drainage organs, and this reduces their function quantitatively and qualitatively. If detoxication, the transport and elimination of metabolic waste products and other forms of ballast becomes difficult, such waste will accumulate in the organism. The result is that the drainage channels, will become blocked, and the humoral milieu deteriorates, finally acquiring pathogenic properties.

It is rather like a swimming pool whose water is not being filtered, whose drain has become clogged; the water will simply get dirtier and dirtier.

The transit mesenchme and RES system may suffer direct damage from causal factors, and they may also be affected indirectly, following the effects of secondary damage on drainage. In this case, mesenchymal function is depressed, lowering natural resistance.

Although there is no doubt the body has a natural resistance to malignant growth processes, if this resistance is reduced, as a result of causal factors and secondary damage, and if there is a carcinogenic disposition, what I describe as a tumour milieu will then exist.

5

And so to the Tumour

TO CREATE THE RIGHT ENVIRONMENT FOR A TUMOUR TO MANIFEST
itself, two essential factors are required, both of them inextricably linked:

1. A lowering of resistance to the point where the body's natural
   defence can no longer cope effectively with malignant cells.
2. The presence of a tumour milieu—the last link in a chain reaction of
   causal factors and secondary damage, together with a specific
   disposition to the disease.

The word milieu is of French derivative and generally means
external environmental conditions. There is also an *internal* milieu.

Numerous researchers have reported the external environment—the
sum total of all the factors surrounding each individual human being—
plays a definite role in the development of cancer. If this were not so,
we could expect cancer to be spread uniformly throughout all parts of
the world.

The opposite is the case. A global study of the disease reveals some
fascinating contradictions. In the United States cancer of the stomach is
statistically low. In South America it is high. In the Irish Republic, skin
and oral cancers are very prevalent. Some eighty miles away in
England, the incidence is dramatically lower; in the case of lip cancer it
is ten times less than in the Republic. France has the greatest incidence of
oral cancers. In Portugal, such cancer is relatively rare. Israel reports a

similar conclusion, but the country has the world's ranking figure for leukaemia. Across the Suez Canal, in Egypt, bladder cancer predominates. In South Africa, the most common cancer is of the skin and prostate. Danish women have the highest rate of breast cancer in the world. In Chile, more women die of cancer of the uterus or stomach than anywhere else.

Why is this? Why is there more cancer of the penis, the liver and back of the mouth in China than there is in Japan? Why does Sweden and Norway have three times as many cases of prostate cancer than does Italy? Why do Italian women have a tendency towards uterine cancer?

Nobody knows for sure why there is this divergence except it is probably caused by local environmental conditions. The West Indian specialist, M. Gilmour, stated that differences can appear in the most circumscribed conditions. In Jamaica she reported breast cancer is almost unknown among the local Chinese population, yet rife among Negroes living on the island. In Fiji, cancerologists found the incidence of cancer of the cervix is far more frequent among Indian women living on the island than among Fijian women. Nobody knows exactly why. There are, however, indications that geographical location and living habits have a certain influence.

Happily, we know somewhat more about the role of the internal milieu as a factor in promoting disease.

Research work into stress has given a new impetus to understanding the internal milieu. The "three factor theory" postulated by Hans Selye, who established the stress syndrome, succinctly explains that illness is always the result of interaction between three quite independent forces:

1. The apparent cause of disease. These are bacteria or any other factors which appear to produce the disease.
2. The factors promoting disease. These can be either internal or external ones, liable to encourage the apparent causal agent. They can produce a disposition towards disease; because of this they are also known as predisposing or "milieu factors".
3. The factors preventing disease. These are the inherent powers of resistance which check the apparent causal agents.

From this can be clearly seen that illness will only occur when (1) and

(2) combine to be more powerful than (3). While (3) remains dominant, no pathological conditions can develop. It is Selye's argument, well substantiated, that there is hardly any causal agent which would be *a priori* a danger to man.

The French physiologist, Claude Bernard (1813–1878) neatly summarized this with his epigram: "The microbe is nothing, environment is all!"

Bernard conducted the first detailed investigation into biology; he found maintenance of a sound internal milieu was a precondition for life. Later, Schade studied the changes in the colloids, molecules and ions which occur with disease; he concluded that the healthy organism endeavours, and is able to maintain, isoionia, isotonia and molecular homoeostasis. This excellent piece of molecular pathology confirmed the old concepts of humoral pathology.

But it is Bernard's work which has made such a valuable contribution to the overall understanding of the internal milieu's function as a disease promoter. He was the first to distinguish between external and internal environmental situations, explaining that the internal milieu is separated from the external milieu by the skin and mucous membranes. The internal milieu is, in turn, divided into the cellular and extracellular, or humoral milieu.

The humoral milieu acts as a carrier for both food and harmful substances from the external environment to the cell, and returns the products of cellular metabolism and catabolism back to the environment. In short, the humoral milieu is a catchment area for this two-way exchange; any change in the external environment, or anything interfering with vital processes in the cell, will automatically involve the humoral milieu. A healthy organism is able to keep the molecular and ionic constitution of the humoral milieu in constant balance by continuously eliminating substances which are unwanted biological ballast. When this ability to maintain homoeostasis is impaired, the molecular constitution of the body fluids will increasingly deviate from what is biologically normal.

The physical state of the blood will also be affected. As the milieu properties of the blood depend on its physical composition, any persisting changes in the acid-base balance, in ionic and electrolyte balance, in blood sugar levels, in serum cholestrol or non-protein nitrogen, will create a tendency towards the development of one kind of disease or another.

In cases of chronic disease, the regulation and diurnal rhythm of the acid-base balance is disturbed. The pH factor of the blood is altered; in cancer patients it becomes more alkaline. Thus indications of alkalosis represent an increased risk of cancer. Changes in the pH factor are usually concurrent with changes in redox potential: a decrease in such reductive capacity is characteristic of many chronic conditions, including cancer. Ionisation and electrical conductivity of the blood are increased if there is chronic disease; the "specific resistance" of the blood, the rho value, is reduced. With cellular damage in an organism there is always a characteristic change in the mineral balance. Serum levels of potassium, magnesium, sodium, zinc, iron and aluminium are usually depressed, while copper serum and calcium tend to be elevated. There is also a tendency for blood sugar to be increased when such damage occurs.

The presence of abnormal constituents is also an indication of a chronic disorder in the metabolism and internal milieu. A completely healthy organism contains only dextrorotatory substances, but they are increasingly found in laevorotatory form in chronic disease. Pathogenic microbes with anaerobic metabolism are up to a thousand times more strongly attracted by compounds with this structure, through chemotaxis, than by the dextro forms of metabolites; consequently in cells subject to toxic damage there is the inevitable parasitic microbes (Gerlach et al.).

The increasing contamination of the organism with laevo forms of metabolites would therefore appear to indicate a particularly serious deterioration of the internal milieu. Denatured proteins may also hasten the process.

In chronic disease a striking change is observed in the appearance, smell, and other characteristics of the body fluids. Hippocrates, around 480 B.C., called it dyscrasia (faulty mixture of the humours); Siegmund termed it "the anarchy of metabolism"; Blumensaat wrote of "a complex metabolic disorder"; others have suggested the term "disturbed homoeostasis". This is the condition which Sir David Smithers, writing in *The Lancet* in 1962, called "disturbed organisation".

With such changes in milieu the organism is predisposed to chronic diseases of all kinds. In Blumensaat's opinion, any chronic metabolic disorder has "the omnipotence for all chronic diseases". This universal potential is no doubt non-specific at the outset; its further development into a rheumatic, uratic, diabetic, carcinogenic or other pathogenic diathesis will, in the final instance, be determined by inherited, toxic, dietetic, or other factors.

Abnormalities in the humoral milieu on the basis of complex metabolic disorders are concomitant not only with biochemical changes but also with changes in the living, solid, constituents of the blood. These changes are discernible under a microscope. If live blood is studied, using dark-ground illumination and a magnification of 1,200, clearly visible are red and white corpuscles and platelets, and minute elements, moving about freely.

In blood from a healthy organism these structures are few and their size so small that they can only be observed by using the dark-ground technique. In cases of chronic diseases, there are many more of them and their size and appearance also tends to be more variable. In addition, larger structures may be present, either within or outside the blood corpuscles. The fact that these structures are found more frequently in cancer patients suggests they are in some way connected with the disease; many investigators have gone so far as to suggest that these protean microbes might be the pathogen responsible for the actual cause of cancer.

The microscopic blood status may be used for the assessment of humoral dyscrasia. The histological diagnosis of dyscrasia is important not just for early diagnosis, but as a relatively simple and reliable aid for assessing the progress of treatment.

When the blood is abnormal, it usually also means the normal colloidal properties have been lost; this can result in an increased tendency to form clots. Researchers have used dried blood to assess the morbid condition of the organism. Similar results can be obtained by using live blood; the process of coagulation and the placement of erythrocytes will still provide relevant diagnostic information.

In healthy blood, the erythrocytes are smooth and round in shape, float freely, lie flat in a single layer, touch only tangentially, do not aggregate or fuse and fibrin fibres appear only singly. In diseased blood, the erythrocytes are vastly different. They have flaccid, wavy outlines, no longer float balloon-like side by side, but show a tendency to become attached to each other. Fibrin fibres are markedly increased.

The distinction I make between first degree dyscrasia, when the morbid symptoms are not very marked; second degree dyscrasia, with medium severe changes; and third degree dyscrasia, with very marked changes.

Another means of studying symptoms of dyscrasia is by examining stained blood. Although the granules are not demonstrable by the usual method of staining, they are well brought out by a method developed by von Brehmer. Dark-ground examination is used, and a magnification of 1,200. Seen against a deep violet background, the erythrocytes appear pale red, pink, or brownish. Granules within or outside them stand out clearly as bright points of light. Assessment is made on the basis of the shape and position of the erythrocytes, and the frequency and appearance of the granules.

In the blood of healthy persons, the erythrocytes lie quite separate from each other; any granules occur singly and are very small.

In the blood of chronically ill persons, the erythrocytes are not separate, and there are granules of many different sizes. The greater the number of large granules, the more serious is the situation. The shape of the granules also permits certain other conclusions to be drawn.

The extent to which the blood has become granular may be taken as an indicator for the unwholesomeness of the humoral milieu. The greater the abnormal changes in the biochemical nature of the blood, the more significant tends to be the change in its microscopic appearance. However, the nature and extent of the changes does not give any definite indication of the disease causing them. Severe arthritis, liver disease, multiple sclerosis and other chronic conditions may involve changes in the blood which cannot in every case be differentiated from the changes seen with malignant disease. Yet the fact that the changes are not specific does not detract from their practical value. Equally, it demonstrates most convincingly that all chronic diseases have a common denominator, the deterioration of the internal milieu.

Microscopic examination of the blood's plasma can provide further evidence of such deterioration.

Treatment by immunotherapy, chemotherapy, and radiotherapy, fragments tumour cells and produces catabolic products. As we have seen, these are toxic and are transported to the organs of detoxication and excretion in the blood and lymph in a process called reintoxication. If reintoxication occurs, microscopic examination will reveal it in the form of coarse or fine granules in the plasma, or by its milky opaqueness.

Pain, fever, and malaise are also general symptoms of reintoxication, and they tend to be more severe the greater the density and granular size of tumour toxins in the plasma. Cancer therapy is therefore much better tolerated if the tumour is dissolved gradually, and only fine granules are produced to be detoxicated and excreted. Causing rapid disintegration of large tumours may result in an extreme degree of reintoxication, and sometimes even present a danger to life. Thus it is important to handle treatment in a way which allows toxic products from the dissolving tumour to remain in manageable proportion; therapy must be adapted to each patient's individual capacity to eliminate them.

If mesenchymal blockage has persisted for a long time, or has been caused, for instance, by X-ray therapy, the tumour often will not respond to immunotherapy. Subsequent basic medical treatment by whole-body therapy may then cause a sudden breach in the blockage, often after weeks or even months. As a result, the blood may be flooded with masses of tumour degradation products—from one hour to the next—causing violent feverish reactions. This flooding always occurs when there are extremely high levels of toxic products in the plasma. The time when such a breakthrough will happen cannot be predicted, and because of this, it is impossible to prevent the consequent febrile reaction.

I have explained my view of how, prior to chronic illness, the body is subject to a complex metabolic disorder which provides the potential for all forms of chronic disease to manifest themselves. The criterion for the potential to form the all-important tumour milieu, or substrate, is fulfilled when the body offers the right conditions for development and propagation to the live oncogenic agent, be it a virus, Mycoplasma, or whatever.

The oncogenic agent is a parasite with anaerobic metabolism and requires quite different metabolites for its food than the normal symbionts in the blood. The higher the concentration of such abnormal metabolites, the more will oncogenic parasites flourish. A tumour milieu, therefore, is a biochemical milieu where cancer parasites or cancer cells find everything they need to live and multiply. If an organism has a tumour milieu, the composition of its humours is "cancer favouring"; the blood contains everything to promote the growth of the cancer cell and of the tumour.

Before discussing the organism's resistance, the body's natural defence system, it is worth repeating two fundamentals:

1. If the body's resistance is intact, it is capable of protecting the body from developing a cancer tumour.
2. If its resistance is weakened to a point leading to immuno-insufficiency, then the way is clear for the formation of a tumour.

It is therefore essential to differentiate between two causal factors in the development of the disease; the intracellular factors which change a normal cell into a cancer cell; and the factors which lower the body's resistance to such an extent that it cannot prevent the formation of a tumour.

Research has shown the body's natural defence potential is a multi-layered structure which, for the sake of clarity, may be summarised as four main functional systems:

1. The adaptive extra-corporal defence zone.
2. The constitutive epithelial defence zone.
3. The constitutive lympho-reticular defence zone.
4. The constitutive reticulo-histiocytary defence zone.
All are closely interrelated and interdependent.

The adaptive extra-corporal defence zone consists of the physiological obligatory microfloras on all epithelial surfaces and has an autonomous defence function as well as a nurse function and is responsible for the development of the basic immunity of the organism. Numerous workers have concluded that multicellular organisms cannot live without a properly functioning symbiotic flora. Further, the other defence zones depend on the eubiotic stability of the microflora of the adaptive extra-corporal zone and its nurse function. If there is a dysbiosis, there is a marked weakening in the organism's overall defence potential.

The epithelial defence zone consists of the skin, and the conjunctival mucous membranes of the eye, of the respiratory tract, of the digestive tract, and of the genito-urinary tract. This zone's functions are absorptive, filtrative, excretory, or defensive. My own clinical experience has shown that the excretory function is of special importance for the elimination of metabolic and oncolytic poisons; a blockage can be largely responsible for metabolic disturbances which affect all the other defence zones and thus indirectly lower the resistance.

The constitutive lympho-reticular defence zone is essentially a back-up system for the epithelial system. It consists of the lympho-epithelial system, the thymus, the Waldeyer tonsillar ring and Peyer's patches of the intestine; the lympho-retothelial system, incorporating the white pulp of the spleen, the lymph nodes and other lymphatic centres; the white bone marrow; the storage endothelia. Its functions are:

1. Phagocytosis, or clearance function.
2. Catalytic induction of antibody production.
3. The production of specific and non-specific antibodies.
4. Detoxification of antigen-antibody complexes and other noxious substances.

When this zone is overstrained, the constitutive reticulo-histiocytary zone is called into action. Until recent years this zone has been neglected in cancer research, but I give it special emphasis because of its great importance for all the defensive processes. This pluripotent mesenchyme, embracing almost half of the body's weight, consists of two systems, each of which preserves its embryonic pluripotency:

1. The reticulo-histiocytary system. This consists of fascia, synoria, ligaments; serous membranes; meninges; non-storing endothelia et al.
2. The ubiquitous interstitial connective tissue; that is, the transitory mesenchyme, the elementary tissue et al.

These two systems perform a number of important functions:

a) Stem-cell function: an omnipotent capacity for forward and backward differentiation.
b) Transitory function: guarantees the mediatorial metabolic processes between epithelial cells and the fibrous tissue, blood, lymph, and control systems.
c) Homoeostatic function: maintains the isotonicity and other components of environmental balance.
d) Storage function: neutralises noxious substances, either by storage or binding.
e) Detoxification function: processes noxious substrates which cannot be reduced by intermediate metabolic mechanisms.
f) Defence function: complements the other systems.

A malignant growth cannot develop unless either one or all of these defence zones are imperilled to the point where the body's resistance is incapable of combating malignant cells, and unable to afford the organism's continued immunity.

The four "main" functional defence systems just described are governed, as are all other organs, by the neuro-hormonic control—which is therefore the fifth link in the defensive mechanism. In any case, resistance is a faculty of the body as a whole. Immunity is transmitted through specific and non-specific substances formed by the immuno-system of the mesenchyme, especially the RES mesenchyme. The extent to which such substances may be produced is dependent on the amount of nervous and hormonal energy available.

The primary objective of the immune system is to try and detect the minutest deviation from the norm in the molecules which are constantly produced by the organism; the immune system maintains its own specific biological identity, not only towards pathogenic organisms and toxins, but also in relation to foreign and degenerated cells—like cancer cells.

If cancer tissue or cancer cells are transplanted into a healthy human being, the result is the same as with transplantation of a healthy organ. Any foreign tissue, be it normal or diseased, is dissolved or rejected by the healthy body's "immune reaction".

In cases of chronic illness, the organism is unable to carry through the proper immune reaction; cancer tissue cannot be quickly enough dissolved. This state of affairs is called immunotolerance, reduced resistance, or lowered defence. It is caused by a deficiency in specific and non-specific immune substances, or an inability on the part of the immune systems to produce such substances in effective form and quantity.

As we have already discussed, the organism is able to mobilise at least four different types of protective substrates against the threat of cancer. It must be emphasised again that each of these needs certain preconditions to become effective. Each defensive factor must be available in such quantity that all antigens arising may be instantly and completely neutralised. The molecular composition of the factor must be such as to guarantee maximum effect. It is also essential that co-factors which may be necessary to make the factor effective, such as magnesium ions, are present in the right form and concentration.

Current scientific thought is that the production of protective factors is a function of the mesenchyme. Non-specific factors are produced in all mesenchymal tissues, but specific defence enyzmes or antibodies are manufactured only by the lymphatic mesenchyme. This mesenchyme derives from the bone marrow, and the stem cells are carried to the thymus by the blood. Thymus hormones convert them to "immunocompetent" lymphocytes, or "immunocytes", and in that state they multiply. The thymus lymphocytes finally migrate to the spleen, the lymph nodes and Peyer's patches on the intestinal wall. The production of antibodies is entirely restricted to those three areas; the thymus itself does not produce them. Its function is to immuno-activate the stem cells brought to it from the bone marrow, and, prob-ably, to store "memory-cells". They are antigen-stimulated immuno-cytes, storing the molecular "information" of antigens and correspond-ing antibodies, so that the latter can immediately be reproduced, if identical antigens invade or arise again.

Like all other organs, mesenchymal tissues may be subject to sec-ondary organic and functional damage, due to many different causal factors. This will obviously also seriously impair their effective poten-tial, and the production of protective factors will decline quantitatively and qualitatively. In such cases, the bone marrow cannot produce enough new stem cells, and those which are produced will have mole-cular defects. The induction of immunoactivity in the thymus will also prove inadequate, and those immunocytes which do reach the spleen, lymph nodes, and Peyer's patches will not be able to function as well as the defence cells of an organism which has not been subject to secondary damage. The reduced defensive powers of the immunocytes are then depressed even further by the lack of activating co-factors and the presence of antienzymes.

A further cause of damage to the soft connective tissues is thought to arise through blockage of drainage channels, stopping the elimination of toxins. Instead, they pass from the humours to the tissues and collect in the basic, or transit tissue, which is so important for resistance. When treatment succeeds in improving drainage, the mesenchyme is cleared of toxic material and this improves resistance.

However, depleted defensive powers may still prove adequate, even if a tumour milieu has already developed in the organism and is providing the soil for the growth and multiplication of oncogenic parasites and cancer cells. Tumour development will still remain checked for as long as non-specific and specific protective factors are produced in sufficient quantity. This situation will only change when, for some reason or other, protective factors are no longer available in effective amounts. When the numbers of newly developed and of destroyed cancer cells are just about even, an unstable condition exists which may easily become a state of permanent imbalance.

Reduced resistance—the relative imbalance between the available potency of defence and the demands made on it—allied with a tumour milieu was called "carcinogenic diathesis", by Beneke in 1880. In 1953, I suggested this should be known as Humoral, or Primary, Precancerosis.

The other precondition for cancer is, of course, the presence of "first cancer cells". These probably do not arise at random somewhere in the body, but in a "weak spot" caused by earlier damage, the site of least resistance. If the milieu is abnormal, and an organ previously damaged continues to suffer further damage, this will cause tissue changes. These need not be malignant to begin with. But if the damaging effects continue they may sooner or later become so. With certain forms of cancer, the actual development of cancer cells or the tumour is undoubtedly preceded by such chronic local tissue changes, usually called local secondary precancerosis.

It is evident, therefore, that this secondary precancerosis can only develop where there is primary precancerosis, a factor naturally to be taken into account when it comes to treatment.

Any chronic illness, however trivial, may develop into precancerosis. Chronic gastritis, or a chronic gastric ulcer, the chronic bronchitis of smokers, chronic cholecystitis or endometritis, may pave the way for cancer of the mucous membranes in the affected area. Benign tumours may develop first in these sites, polyps for example, or papillomata, and if the irritation causing the damage continues these may progressively develop into malignancies.

Nevertheless, it appears in the majority of cases that the malignant tumour arises *directly* on the mucous membrane previously subjected to chronic damage, and is *not* preceded by a benign neoplasma.

Malignant tumours never develop, and this includes occupational tumours, unless there has first been a state of chronic inflammation (Becker). Whether inflammation leads to proliferation depends on the duration of it, on the local situation, on whether causal factors persist, on an increasing inability to eliminate toxins, and on the trigger factor.

Every cancer has its "precancer" (Virchow). As a rule this, too, produces few or no symptoms, and thus often remains undiagnosed. Consequently, most malignant tumours unfortunately seem to arrive unexpectedly.

Whether and when primary precancerosis progresses to malignancy after secondary precancerosis, depends on a number of factors. In some cases, a physical or psychological trigger coincides with an advanced disposition to the disease and a tumour is produced quite quickly. In others, the transition from benign to malignant development in a previously damaged site is a very gradual one, over a long period of time, and quite unnoticeable.

As stress results in immuno-depression, the release of increased amounts of stress hormones causes limitation and inhibition of functions in the mesenchymal organs of defence.

In a healthy person, even very severe stress presents no real danger providing it is only temporary. But if there is chronic illness, the resulting immuno-depression may have fatal consequences. Any acute stress situation will for a time open up the barriers of the body's defences against inherited and residual toxicoses, against foci of infection, particularly in the teeth and tonsils, and also the barriers set up against toxins entering at the epithelial surfaces of, for instance, the intestine. Thus, during stress, the many different and highly dangerous toxins normally held back by these barriers will spread unchecked in the organism. They will be able to produce their toxic effects in all tissues, affecting the entire organism, in the cellular and the humoral milieu.

Further, the secondary damage already present—including damage to the defence systems—will inevitably be aggravated; toxins becoming established in the body will considerably increase the demands made on the defence system. At the same time they will also clog the mesenchyme, causing a further reduction, and finally blockage, of its defensive powers. The more intense the immuno-depression due to stress, and the greater its duration, the sooner this will happen.

Physical trauma—injury or bruising—may also serve as the trigger factor if it involves a weak point produced by earlier damage, or else gives rise to one. If primary precancerosis is fully developed, and if, for instance, there are nodular lesions in the breast, bruising may induce the development of breast cancer.

Tumour growth only occurs where there are cancer cells. The

first growth—the primary tumour—tends to develop in that part of the body affected by precancerosis, where the "first cancer cells" have arisen.

From this primary tumour, cancer cells migrate, reaching all parts of the organism via the blood and lymphatic channels. Under certain conditions they may form secondary tumours, or metastases.

If the primary tumour has been removed and a new tumour forms, this new growth is called a recurrence. If the new tumour appears in the same site as the primary tumour, it is a local recurrence; if it appears in the vicinity of the primary tumour, it is called a regional recurrence; if the new manifestation takes the form of metastases, it is called a metastatic recurrence.

Malignant disease may also occur in generalised, systemic form from the beginning, for instance as:

a) myelosis—malignant disease of the bone marrow;
b) lymphadenosis—malignant disease of the lymphatic systems;
c) lymphogranulomatosis (Hodgkin's disease)—a condition involving malignant changes in the lymph nodes.

The characteristic features of malignant tumours, according to K. H. Bauer, are:

1. autonomous growth,
2. unrestrained proliferative and destructive capacity,
3. ability to produce metastases,
4. ability to produce recurrences for as long as residual, undestroyed cancer tissue remains in the body.

As a rule, there are no symptoms or signs, subjective or clinical, to mark the stages in the development of cancer which precedes the manifestation of the tumour. Even the early stages of actual tumour formation do not usually produce symptoms which raise an alarm. This situation must be held responsible for the fact that two-thirds of malignant conditions are diagnosed so late that surgery and irradiation are ineffectual. Different forms of cancer show tremendous variation in progress, but this unnoticeable, insidious, onset is common to them all.

As a rule, pain will only be caused by malignant neoplasms when nerves in the area suffer damage from pressure or infiltration. In most cases, no pain is felt during the very early stages of tumour growth.

Ulcers refusing to heal, on the skin, the tongue, mucous membranes of the mouth, the pharynx, the larynx, the uterus or internal organs, may be early symptoms of malignant neoplasms. The development of a crater at the base of an ulcer is characteristic of cancer of the stomach, intestine, and air passages.

When a tumour ulcerates or infiltrates other tissues, blood vessels are opened up, and this results in haemorrhage. Abnormal uterine bleeding, for example, may be the first symptom of cancer of the uterus; tumours of the urinary tract may announce their presence through blood in the urine; visible traces of blood in the stools may be the first indication of neoplastic lesions in the colon. Blood from tumours in the small intestine and stomach usually remains concealed.

If a tumour develops in the walls or anywhere near one of the hollow organs, as it increases in size it naturally causes a narrowing of the organ, so that passage within it is impeded. Neoplasms of the oesophagus may make themselves felt through difficulties in swallowing; tumours of the stomach may interfere with normal emptying of the organ; tumours of the intestine may cause retention of stool, and sometimes even complete obstruction.

Rapidly growing tumours often cause the destruction or penetration of adjoining organs. A stomach cancer may penetrate into the large intestine or pancreas, cancer of the oesophagus into the air passages or aorta.

From the above descriptions of the local symptoms of cancer, it can be seen that when the disease is first detected, it is usually the complications produced by the tumour which are diagnosed.

But now let us turn to the general symptoms. As we know, the constituents of the cancer cell and its metabolic products are highly toxic. Because of this, tumour growth is always concomitant with continuous poisoning, intoxication, of the host organism. Exhaustion, loss of energy, and other non-specific general symptoms are the result.

The continuous poisoning through the tumour is taken even further when tumour tissue disintegrates, causing reintoxication of the body with toxic amines. The emaciation and deterioration of the body of tumour patients must be ascribed primarily to this intoxication and reintoxication. If the intake and utilisation of food are also reduced, these conditions develop all the more rapidly.

There are patients who, even at very advanced tumour stages, show no generalised symptoms whatsoever, and are apparently in such "good" general condition that the truth is concealed. Their body does not react to the disease, it remains silent in the face of all provocation, until finally proliferation grows rampant and the advanced condition, usually fatal, is manifest.

They are perhaps the most unfortunate of all. For had they produced symptoms at an earlier stage, they would probably have gone to their doctor. Assuming he was conversant with the latest forms of cancer therapy, it is possible they might have been saved, if not by surgery, radiotherapy, or chemotherapy—by combining whole-body therapy and immunotherapy.

6

Immunotherapy: The Fourth Weapon

SOME EARLY OBSERVERS HAVE CLAIMED THAT UNEXPLAINED REMISSIONS from cancers were due to an immune response by the patient. It is only now that we are in a position to substantiate such observations by laboratory methods and to make rational use of immunological procedures for the prevention, diagnosis and treatment of cancer. It is clear there is a vital role for this modality of cancer treatment, immunotherapy. That branch of medical science deals with immunity to disease; immunity being a state of resistance to a specific disease, and immunotherapy the treatment of that disease through immunological principles.

One further point needs to be added. Immunotherapy appears to have a far better chance of success within the framework of whole-body therapy. In my own clinical experience, results have been obtained in a significant percentage of cases. For over twenty years I have documented my experience and results with some eight thousand cancer cases treated by such methods. The response was frequently a heartening prolonging of life.

I believe there are four reasons why immunotherapy has not, until now, received greater emphasis. It was eclipsed by the advent of radiation therapy, and later chemotherapy. Dramatic responses to microbial vaccines were somewhat unpredictable. No standard laboratory procedure was initially available for assaying the anti-tumour activity of various microbial products. No explanation of the mechanism of action was immediately forthcoming; this made it

difficult to devise research programmes which would explain the action
of microbial products on the course of cancer, and so provide clues as to
how such treatment might be more generally applied.

Since the mid 1950s, following the elucidation of the basic rules of
tissue transplantation and the development of inbred strains of animals
—two prerequisites for immunological research to progress—there has
been a burgeoning interest in cancer immunotherapy. Even so it still
appears to many doctors to be the most complex and incomprehensible
of all the disciplines concerned with managing the disease. Compared
with other treatments, immunotherapy is wrapped in mystery, has a
language all its own, and it has been said that even immunologists
sometimes do not precisely understand each other.

This is partly because "modern" immunology is still very new; it
will be 1980 before it celebrates the twenty-fifth anniversary of what
that distinguished Australian immunologist, G. J. V. Nossal, has
rightly termed "the golden second age of immunology".

Nevertheless as the evidence accumulates, the conviction grows that
some human cancers, like many animal cancers, are produced by viruses.
Final proof has still to come because such viruses frequently assume a
concealed form in cancer cells and thus cannot be readily demonstrated.
Instead their presence is revealed by immunological means which
detect the antigens which are the hallmark of the unseen virus; antigens,
in immunological terms, are any substance which the body recognises
as foreign and to which it responds by making antibodies.

Using reactions between antibodies in the patient and the antigens in
his tumour cells, the virus that caused the tumour can be identified
even though the tumour itself does not contain a "complete" virus.
Current work with human sarcomas, a type of cancer, provides an
excellent example. So far it has not been possible to constantly demonstrate a virus in these tumours. But the serum of many of these sarcoma
patients contains an antibody that reacts with the antigen found in
human sarcomas which is thought to belong to a *causative* virus.
Similar and related findings are being now made with other neoplasia
in man. The major and immediate challenge is to identify the antigens
involved and so discover which cancers are related to one another, and
are caused by the same virus.

Today there is general agreement that any microbial agents play
their part in the emergence of cancer. The last decades have seen
intensive investigations into what kind of microbe is responsible.

Some researchers argue that the virus itself is the actual cause of the disease; others say that virus-like organisms—mycoplasms—are responsible. Various aspects indicate that it might be one and the same oncogenic agent which occurs in both and even in bacteria-like forms. This is a phenomenon known as pleo-morphism.

The finding of antigens in tumours provides a new rationale for early diagnosis of cancer. Some of these antigens may appear in the blood where they can be detected by the production of their respective antibodies. The development of rapid and sensitive assays of such antigens, as and when they are discovered, is important in successful early diagnosis. This is just one avenue of immunological research which shows the "second coming" of immunology is still in an ascendent phase.

To understand more fully this rebirth of interest in immune mechanisms we must go back to that first golden age of immunology.

An English physician, Edward Jenner (1749–1823) fathered immunology when he inoculated an eight-year-old boy with fluid from a cowpox pustule in a successful attempt to give him resistance against the more virulent smallpox. Jenner knew nothing about the immune system, but he had recognised that milkmaids who frequently came in contact with cows suffering from cowpox seldom contracted smallpox. Jenner had, of course, found no answer to cancer, but down the years a hypothesis grew that somehow the natural immunological defences of the body did respond against disease agents; only when the body defences were overrun did a disease rampage to its often deadly conclusion.

It was not until the 1850s—after Louis Pasteur discovered the existence of bacteria and propounded the germ theory of disease—that scientists began to seriously suspect the body had a mechanism for identifying and combating disease agents. The search began for an effective immunotherapy agent to reinforce the ailing natural defences.

Christmas Eve, 1891, was a dramatic turning point in the history of immunology. In Berlin, in a clinic, a little German girl lay dying from diphtheria. She was in a state of shock and her attending doctor was in despair. By chance that great German scientist, E. A. von Behring, was working late in the city's university clinic when he heard of the child's plight. A year before he had been one of the co-discoverers of a substance called *Antikörper;* this appeared in the bloodstream after infections and animal experiments had proved it was capable of neutralising poisons. In a further experiment, von Behring had successfully inoculated a sheep with diphtheria antigen. Late on Christmas Eve, 1891, he decided to make the dying child the world's first known immunological guinea pig. He injected the little girl with some of the sheep's serum—thus creating *passive* immunisation, the transfer of antibodies produced by one animal or person to the bloodstream of another. By Christmas morning the child began to revive. Ten years later von Behring's courageous decision helped win him the first Nobel prize in medicine, for the child's ultimate total recovery signified an immunological milestone. In effect it was the first occasion in which medical science had cured an acute infectious disease.

In 1891, on the other side of the world from Berlin, in America, a gifted surgeon, William Coley, had also begun conducting a series of experiments after observing the beneficial effects of certain infections on his cancer patients. He injected selected patients with mixed bacterial toxins to induce responses that might change the course of the malignancy. Coley, not fully understanding the immunological process he had started, managed to arrest the course of cancer. In 1893 he had injected his toxin into a young boy with inoperable, incurable cancer. Coley's courage—for if he had failed he might well have faced professional stricture—was rewarded with a notable success: the boy's tumour regressed over a few days, finally disappearing after a few months. All told, Coley treated some four hundred and eighty-three further patients. In *each case* there was a clear clinical improvement. A later assessment of his records shows that two hundred and eighty-three of those patients survived for a period ranging from five to seventy-two years longer than their medical prognosis had indicated. Coley was far ahead of his time, probably one reason why his work went unrecognised.

Nevertheless, immunology was gradually assuming the form of an accepted science as it became increasingly clear that the body's power to resist could have a scientific explanation. Doctors began to realise that, in the case of infectious diseases, the internal milieu and the resistance were far more important in deciding the course of an illness than the pathogen.

While Coley inoculated his toxins, a German researcher, Scheuerlen, had already reported in 1886 that cancer cells contained a specific motile cancer bacillus which could be grown and transferred, causing tumours in hitherto healthy animals. His finding played a significant part in the entire future of cancer research: it heralded the hunt for a cancer-causing pathogen which continues to this day. It also paved the way for the view that if a micro-organism was partly responsible for the development of cancer, that only confirmed the concept of cancer as a systemic disease.

From this it was possible to further postulate that, as with any infection, when the body's resistance and the internal milieu were disturbed, those micro-organisms caused cancer. This idea provided a satisfactory solution to many of the problems which had faced nineteenth-century scientists in cancer research. It allowed for a clearer picture to emerge as to why everybody did not develop cancer—and why one patient suffered metastases and another did not.

Various doctors continued to confirm the earlier work of Jenner by observing that tumours regressed or even disappeared when concurrent diseases developed, such as gangrene, smallpox, and erysipelas: if the concurrent infection caused a high temperature, this often had a beneficial effect on the malignant process.

Step by immunological step the theoretical aspects of bodily defences were probed—and proven. In 1891, Adamkiewicz, addressing the Imperial Academy of Sciences in Vienna, reported regression of malignant tumours had been achieved with a substance called *cancroin*, which he had obtained from cancer cells. In subsequent years he published an impressive list of cures claimed for this drug. In 1895 attempts at passive immunisation were made by Richet and Héricourt, this time in the treatment of cancer. They used serum from an animal previously inoculated with cancer cells. They reported that improvement occurred in some cases, often with a marked reduction in tumour size. Further success in this field was reported in 1902 by E. von Leyden, F. Blumenthal and C. O. Jensen. That year, a French surgeon, Doyen, also announced he had successfully treated superficial and deeper-seated tumours with a vaccine prepared from what he termed "micrococcus neoformans". Using attenuated cultures of the pathogen, he claimed forty-two out of two hundred and forty-two patients, most of them designated "incurable". He reported his findings to the International Medical Congress in Madrid in 1903.

That year Paul Ehrlich earned himself a place in the expanding literature of immunology by publishing a remarkable series of reports of cures in animal cancers. Today, it is fashionable in some quarters to decry Ehrlich's work as being "completely valueless because of inadequate experimental methods". In 1970, Robert Baldwin, director of the British Empire Cancer Campaign Research laboratories in Nottingham, dismissed Ehrlich as a man working in "a background of almost total ignorance of the science of transplantation immunology ... (that) produced an atmosphere of complete chaos and the early hopes that vaccination would lead to a cure for cancer were replaced by a total condemnation of this approach".

G. V. Nossal, a world authority on immunology, prefers to see Ehrlich, as I do, in a kinder light; to acknowledge that he was the giant of German science in the early part of this century. Ehrlich was a superb chemist with a profound interest in biology; the microbial world and the host-parasite relationship fascinated him, and no aspect more so than the body's capacity to form antibodies. His dream was to combine chemistry and biology into rational treatments for infectious diseases by constructing "golden bullets" which would move in the bloodstream, exerting a toxic action on microbes while leaving the host tissue untouched. His discovery of arsenical drugs for the treatment of syphilis is a classic example of how his dream was partially fulfilled.

His was the first coherent theory of antigen formation, formulated in 1897. The essence of Ehrlich's "side-chain" theory was that cells had chemical groupings, or side-chains, some of which, by sheer chance, would fit to the chemical groupings of the antigen. This would naturally interfere with whatever was the normal function of the side-chain in the cell, allowing the cell to regenerate more side-chains. Ehrlich claimed the antitoxins represent nothing more than the side-chains reproduced in excess during regeneration and are therefore pushed off from the protoplasm—thus to exist in a free state.

That may indeed, by modern standards, be rather imprecise. It may also be true to say that Ehrlich may not have made any *direct* major contribution to cancer etiology. But, like Nossal, I believe his name will forever be enshrined as one of the great father-figures of immunology.

While Ehrlich was propounding his antigen theory, another German doctor, O. Schmidt, was arousing considerable interest in his work on a specific immunotherapy for cancer. In 1903 he achieved regression of tumours by this means—the first man to do so. For the next two years the scientific journals of England and Germany contained numerous papers by Schmidt describing his methods and the results he obtained with his preparation, *Antimeristem*. In 1911 he reported on the treatment of 304 cancer patients: 192 responded; in 86 cases the tumour regressed completely and he claimed 28 cures. It was, by any account, an astonishing success record.

Between 1910 and 1920, Nebél, in Lausanne, using a vaccine for treating incurable patients, almost identical to Schmidt's, reported that he had successfully combined immunotherapy with homoeopathic treatment to improve the internal milieu. He particularly stressed the importance of "canalisation", i.e. drainage. Without the body having an effective "drainage system"—seldom present in cancer patients—immunotherapy would fail. He gave detailed descriptions of how canalisation could be restored.

Over the years, one piece of research followed another to show that a badly functioning immune system, or the absence of one, left the body virtually defenceless against infection from within or without. In passing, more than one eminent scientist bluntly stated that the principles upon which cancer research had hitherto been based were wrong, and that the disease must be tackled from quite a different approach if there was to be more effective methods of treatment.

It is a view I have urged in a lifetime of clinical experience in treating cancer.

The learned journals of the 1920/30s are filled with arguments that cancer, in immunological terms, must be regarded as a disease of the whole organism. This view was supported by such researchers as Professor Franz Gerlach in Vienna, who demonstrated Mycoplasma-type organisms in carcinomas and sarcomas.

Since 1958 Professor Gerlach has been Head of the Microbiological Research Unit at my clinic. He has filled the gaps in the chain of evidence relating to the role of Mycoplasma organisms in the development of malignant tumours. In a series of laboratory experiments he grew a pure culture of Mycoplasma organisms obtained from tumours; produced various types of malignant tumours and leukaemia in animals by giving depot inoculations of virulent pure cultures; achieved the regression of malignant tumours in animals and humans by means of a vaccine made from attenuated Mycoplasma cultures.

After ten years' research Gerlach first published his theory about Mycoplasma in 1937. He showed that all human and animal tumours contained a virus-like substance. He was ahead of his time. Few oncologists of that day could comprehend his theory. Later, in the post-war years, researchers followed, and expanded, the trail Gerlach had pioneered twenty years earlier. They referred to Mycoplasma as bacteroids or pleuro-pneumonia-like organisms.

While their research continued, Gerlach produced a vaccine and published proof of its effectiveness against cancer. The vaccine causes the organism to produce anti-Mycoplasma antibodies. These attack only malignant tissues, whether primary or secondaries without damaging any healthy cells or organs.

Some twelve thousand miles away from Gerlach's laboratories in Bavaria, another respected researcher, virologist Sir Frank Macfarlane Burnet, was, in the 1950s, taking another great step forward for immunology—and mankind. In his laboratories in Melbourne, Australia, Burnet was applying his intellect to a question that forty years before had fascinated Ehrlich: recognition in the immune system; how do the lymphocytes recognise "self" from "non-self"; how does the body rid itself of worn-out or unwanted constituents arising within it, such as ageing red cells, *without* an apparent immune response—while dealing with foreign matter from the external milieu largely through antibody formation?

Burnet believed the whole question of self-recognition was crucial to the full understanding of antibody formation. After much experimental work with animals, Burnet theorised that the body manages to cope with the enormous range of pathogenic microbes by a complex system, whose main agents are the lymphocytes, which are produced by the so-called "stem-cells" of the bone marrow, the mushy, reddish substance that produces blood components.

Once formed, the lymphocytes develop into two distinct types of cells, T and B cells, each playing an important role in immune response. Those that pass through the thymus area become T cells, the main agents of that phenomenon known as "cell-mediated immunity". T cells are responsible for maintaining the body's biological uniqueness by rejecting foreign matter. When such organisms threaten the body, the macrophages react like a nuclear early warning system. Coming in contact with them, they trigger off an immunological alarm, despatching T cells to isolate and chemically destroy this foreign matter.

When the body receives a red alert it is being attacked, B cells are automatically stimulated to produce antibodies which affix themselves to the enemies making them far more susceptible to swifter destruction. This process is achieved by dissolving them into chemical components which are recycled by the body and excreted as waste.

In the middle of the 1950s, the period that marked the "second coming" of the golden age of immunolgoy, Burnet and Dr. Lewis Thomas, who had just assumed the position of President of the Sloan-Kettering Cancer Center, New York, suggested there was a relationship between the immune system and cancerous growth. They argued that in addition to protecting the body from foreign intruders, the immune system also functioned as a "police force", to prevent the survival and multiplication of abnormal cells. They postulated that in the organism where cells are continually replicating themselves, every day must see the production of thousands of abnormal, genetically different and potentially cancerous cells. Ordinarily, the immune system would recognise and destroy them before they divided.

But when the defence mechanism is weakened, for *any* reason, it is unable to fulfil this task. The malignant cells multiply, reproduce themselves at an alarming rate, invade normal tissue, and eventually kill the host. From all this it is clear, as Dr. Robert Good, the present Director of Sloan-Kettering says, that Man lives in a sea of micro-organisms; the immune system is his licence to survive.

Good and his research team reported in 1973 that they had observed a high correlation between cancer and the so-called immunodeficiency diseases which leave their victims unable to resist infection. Such a finding is consistent with my own clinical experience.

Reactivating immunity is never easy. But, as we shall now see, there are today definite immunological avenues open to stimulate the natural resistance.

Specific active immunotherapy is defined as the stimulation of im-mune reactions directed against tumour-associated antigens; non-specific active immunotherapy is the general stimulation of the host's immune reactions by "adjuvants" (Mathé).

Put another way, immunology allows for two courses of action. Essentially they are: specific immunisation; and augmenting the immune responses.

Specific immunisation works on a well-tried principle. Once a particular cancer antigen has been identified it is administered under conditions most favourable for the induction of an immune response that will destroy cancer cells bearing that antigen. This is really no more than an extension of the standard vaccination technique against any infectious disease. The effectiveness of this approach in cancer treatment has still to be fully achieved. As we have already discussed the great problem is a total understanding of how immunity resistance can be transferred from one individual to another. This is most important for cancer patients with unexplained defects in their immune capacity. Again, research has shown that the three accepted modes of cancer therapy in different degrees all suppress the host's natural immune capacity. A special goal in the treatment of patients who have undergone surgery, radiotherapy and chemotherapy is to try and supply them with "preformed" resistance in the form of immune cells or sub-cellular material, a procedure called "adoptive" immunisation.

Augmenting the immune responses is also complicated by the fact that the immune capacity of even a healthy individual is not inexhaustible. It is now known that the ability to maintain an effective peak of resistance that responds to antigens declines with age and is adversely affected by any serious illness. Just as there are many drugs and other agents used in cancer therapy which depress the functions of the body's natural resistance, so there are others which raise the immune response, or make existing immunity more effective. It has been clearly shown, in animal experiments, that immune responses can be boosted. The most effective agents for doing this are products derived from bacteria and fungi; animals treated with such vaccines are more resistant to certain types of cancer as well as to bacterial and viral infections.

To understand the practical applications of immunotherapy we need to have a sound grasp of the functions of the immune system. Some of the facts may be very elementary. I make no apology for that. A substantial foundation of detailed knowledge of how things work before they go wrong is essential in all aspects of medicine.

We shall begin by trying to answer that most basic of all questions: what is resistance?

There is no one answer to that question. For a start there are two kinds of *passive* resistance: structural resistance; and metabolic resistance.

With structural resistance, as the name implies, the structure of a cell can hinder the introduction of foreign matter by superficial epithelia. Metabolic resistance comes into play after the invasive foreign cells have penetrated the structural resistance. To continue surviving beyond that point the intruders need to lock on the other metabolites and enzymes. Metabolic resistance ensures this does not happen.

Next, there is *active* resistance, the capacity of an organism to stop a microbial invasion by counter-attacking in the hope that the intruders will be destroyed before they are able to gain an infectious foothold in the body.

The biological importance of such defence processes are manifold:

1. They protect the body from bombardment by a variety of elements in the external environment which have mutagenic potency. This protection is extended to cover the side-effects of cosmic radiation: in any one year the human body is subjected and penetrated by at least 10,000,000 high-energy ultra corpuscles of cosmic radiation. The defence system ensures that this potentially lethal attack is effectively combated. Cosmic radiation is only one of innumerable and equally dangerous mutagenics that the defence system heads off.

2. The core of this system is its ability to identify each abnormal cell and to destroy it by a process called "homograft immunity", a means we have already discussed in which the system distinguishes between "self" and "non-self" cells.

3. Once more it becomes clear that whether a tumour will develop depends totally upon the body's defence system. Impairment to a certain degree leads to the soil for cancer to manifest itself. This is called "defect immunopathy"—the inability of the body to provide antigenic stimulation on its own accord.

The pathology of defect immunopathy is based on structural and functional damage within the immune-competent systems of the body. This damage is found in the thymus, the spleen, the bone marrow, the lymph-nodes, Peyer's patches of the intestines and all other lympho-reticular areas. Damage also appears as functional defects in immuno-competent migrant cells. Causal factors for this damage include: malnutrition, stress, chemical toxins, residual toxicosis, dysbacteria, prenatally acquired deficiency diseases etc.

Immuno-insufficiency can be managed by immunotherapy in a significant number of cases. But there is a long way to go before we can say that immunology holds the answer to the problems of cancer. Nossal has pointed out several major difficulties in any immunothera-peutic approach. There is still the need to settle once and for all whether human cancers are virally induced, chemically induced, or even whether they exhibit tumour-specific antigens. We know that malignant cells are especially prone to *further* mutation which may follow the original one and might be associated with a changing antigenic pattern. Nossal argues that in all probability, any vaccination procedure using tissue from another human would cause more antibody formation against the foreign histo-compatibility antigens than against the much weaker tumour-specific antigens. Finally, there is a strange phenomenon known as tumour enhancement when, after active immunotherapy, the tumour actually increases in size, for reasons not yet understood. What is known is that, in these unusual cases, for some reason the organism does not respond properly by producing the required anti-bodies—or at least not in sufficient numbers—and instead it uses this potential for purposes not intended.

With this note of very necessary caution we can now look briefly at the practical application of immunotherapy in cancer treatment at the time of writing.

Active immunisation stimulates the endogenous reactions by vaccination with living, sometimes attenuated, tumour cells derived from human or animal tumours, or vaccination with living, but sometimes attenuated oncogenetic parasites from the same sources. This can be performed with autologous, homologous or heterologous vaccines.

Autologous vaccines can be produced from either tumour extracts or the blood of patients receiving these vaccines. Homologous vaccines such as those produced by Franz Gerlach, are prepared from the blood or tumours of other cancer patients. Heterologous vaccines are prepared from animal tumours.

While each of these vaccines can be therapeutically effective it cannot always be determined beforehand which vaccine is capable of giving an optimal result in any particular case. My own clinical experience shows it is advisable to switch from one vaccine to another when the desired results are not forthcoming. There are indications that organ-homologous vaccines are more effective than those prepared from other sources. The effect of an active-specific immunotherapy can sometimes be markedly improved by the simultaneous use of large doses of a non-specific vaccine, such as BCG (for Bacillus Calmette-Guerin, after the Frenchmen who developed it).

In the United States, Lloyd Old has done valuable work on the practical application of BCG for stimulating the host reaction in neoplasia.

Georges Mathé, the French cancer researcher, has reported that while BCG is, of course, not a specific anti-cancer drug as such, it does indeed appear to be a powerful immuno-potentiator, a tool for stimulating the immune system. When injected into patients who either have a natural or acquired immunity to tuberculosis, it has the effect of jogging their immunological "memory" of the disease and so produces a swift and generalised immune response.

In cases of cancer BCG is directed, whenever possible, into the cancer lesions. This procedure triggers a complex immune response which enables the body's defence system, to destroy cancer cells. Mathé has been using BCG since 1964 as part of a "double-barrelled approach" to treating patients with acute lymphoid leukaemia. In America, Donald Morton of U.C.L.A. has been using BCG to activate the immune systems in cases of malignant melanoma. Edmund Klein of Roswell Park Memorial Institute in Buffalo was reported in 1973 to have achieved immune reaction by using BCG against malignant melanoma, mycosis fungoids and other types of cancer.

Passive immunisation is created in patients by injecting them with antibodies which have been prepared from repeated vaccination of healthy animals, or human beings. This passive immunisation can destroy tumour cells to a certain degree. Similar immunity can be created by the use of non-specific substrates like Interferon, and several further virus inactivating complementary factors.

Inteferon was discovered in 1957 by Isaacs in England, who showed that Interferon production or release is stimulated by viruses, bacteria and other micro-organisms as well as of course by bacterial vaccines, fungal extracts and certain synthetic polysaccarides, poly-inosite compounds and similar substrates. Interferon is a remarkable substance, acting in one to four hours, much faster than other immune mechanisms. It has been shown to have a clear anti-tumour activity. Steroids and chemotherapy interfere with the production of Interferon.

As we have already seen, the lowered resistance of a cancer patient's organism is mainly the result of a deficiency in defence-active immunocytes. By injecting leucocytes of the same group—or cells from the spleen, thymus or bone marrow—of healthy donors, this deficiency can be rectified, especially if the donor has been immunised by repeated vaccination with oncogenetic substrates. This procedure is known as *adoptive* immunotherapy.

All these immunological methods are designed to supply or produce in the organism protective substances which specifically destroy cancer cells. Their mode of action is the following:

1. All presenting cancer foci can be inhibited and gradually stimulated to regress.
2. Roving cancer cells can be destroyed and further metastases prevented.
3. Toxic tumour proteins are partially metabolised into excretable compounds.

Whole-body therapy represents a preparation of the host for immunotherapy to realise its maximum effect. This varies to a marked degree from patient to patient. Such preparation is essential because immunotherapy leads to a disintegration of cancer cells and the production in the host of highly toxic metabolites causing reintoxication. This manifests itself either as a local reaction in the tumour site, with pain and inflammation as the attendant symptoms, or as a febrile general reaction. The greater the amounts of metabolites transported into the blood stream, the more noticeable are these effects. The reactive swelling in the tumour site can sometimes be so intensive that adjacent cavities can temporarily be constricted. In intestinal tumours the intestinal passage can be blocked; brain tumours can be accompanied by severe headaches and increased intracranial pressure.

Specific measures can be applied to try and offset these unpleasant effects. Firstly, great care must be taken to use only the smallest possible vaccine dosage, and to increase it very slowly. Secondly, the detoxifying potency of the liver and connective tissue must be supported by suitable preparations. Thirdly, the excretory functions of the drainage and valve organs must be stimulated.

Even so, since the individual response of a patient can suddenly change due to any of several reasons, excessive reactions to immunotherapy cannot always be prevented. But they can be generally overcome by using suitable antiphlogistics, such as antihistamines, calcium, magnesium et al.

It is also worth remembering that while active immunotherapy can enforce an increased activity in diseased connective tissue, such tissue cannot be regenerated simultaneously by these measures.

In the 1970s immunology as a cancer therapy has received a considerable amount of publicity. As Mathé says the reason for this lies not only in the failure of other methods of therapy available today, and therefore the need for a complementary treatment but also in the mode of action of active immunotherapy which, unlike other procedures, can kill the last remaining malignant cell, so extending life.

The future of immunotherapy is going to depend on several research programmes:

1. Research into tumour-associated antigens in human cancers and the immunological reactions that they excite.
2. Research into new adjuvants. In this respect there is a need for developing screening programmes.
3. Research into the preparation of specific vaccines.

From all this may indeed come the longed-for hope of producing a lasting immunity in all cancer patients. Like G. J. V. Nossal, I also share the hope and belief, that, in the end, immunological techniques will assume a role, and perhaps the dominant role, in the fight against cancer.

But whatever immunological measures are taken—whether it is stimulation, passive or active immunisation—one factor should always be considered: every effort must be made to ensure all the body's defence mechanisms are mobilised and normalised.

7

A System of Treatments

THE WHOLE-BODY APPROACH TO THE PRACTICAL MANAGEMENT OF cancer is a combination of two distinct therapies which complement each other.

One is a basic causal therapy to reactivate the host's natural defence. This therapy must correspond in every single measure with the pathological path leading to the disease; it must be modified to suit each patient.

The other is a specific tumour therapy aimed at eliminating the local symptom of the disease, the tumour, by the conventional methods, including the latest weapon in this armoury, immunotherapy.

This combined treatment regime may be summarised as on page 107.

Both the basic causal therapy and the tumour therapy are carried out simultaneously.

The aim of the basic therapy is:

1. Elimination of all causal factors, such as dental and tonsilar foci and fields of neural disturbance, abnormal intestinal flora, faulty diet, exogenous chemical and physical factors, and psychic stress.
2. Treatment of secondary damage and tumour milieu to restore normal functions of organs and organ systems. This can be achieved by general measures, and by substitution.

106

COMBINATION THERAPY OF CANCER (ISSELS 1953)

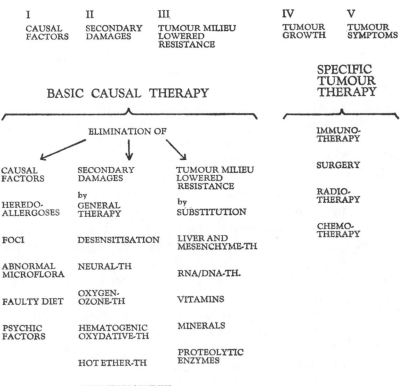

I	II	III		IV	V
CAUSAL FACTORS	SECONDARY DAMAGES	TUMOUR MILIEU LOWERED RESISTANCE		TUMOUR GROWTH	TUMOUR SYMPTOMS

BASIC CAUSAL THERAPY

SPECIFIC TUMOUR THERAPY

ELIMINATION OF

CAUSAL FACTORS	SECONDARY DAMAGES	TUMOUR MILIEU LOWERED RESISTANCE	IMMUNO-THERAPY
	by	by	SURGERY
HEREDO-ALLERGOSES	GENERAL THERAPY	SUBSTITUTION	
			RADIO-THERAPY
FOCI	DESENSITISATION	LIVER AND MESENCHYME-TH	CHEMO-THERAPY
ABNORMAL MICROFLORA	NEURAL-TH	RNA/DNA-TH.	
FAULTY DIET	OXYGEN-OZONE-TH	VITAMINS	
PSYCHIC FACTORS	HEMATOGENIC OXYDATIVE-TH	MINERALS	
	HOT ETHER-TH	PROTEOLYTIC ENZYMES	
	AUTO-HORMONE-TH		
	REHYDRATION		
	FEVER		

These basic treatments, like all scientifically based therapies, are tailored to meet the needs of individual patients. Some of them will be familiar to every doctor; some may well be new. That would be no reason to reject their usefulness in favourably influencing the course of cancer, to offer even the "incurables" a real extension of valuable living and, sometimes a cure.

Every effort should be made to desensitise the organism which has been sensitised by causal factors. Beneficial results are obtained by injection of autovaccines prepared from teeth and tonsillar extracts, as well as from pathogenic coli bacteria and the administration of Spenglersan etc.

Neural Therapy enables the distant effects of a primary focus to be made asymptomatic. In the next chapter I shall discuss teeth and tonsil foci—primary foci—and argue for their elimination. But, as we shall see, even after removal of such primary foci, it is still necessary to treat the distant symptoms.

Every cell and every organ has an energy potential in proportion to its redox potential. In a focus, this redox potential has broken down; the cells have become depolarised and are in a state of constant, pathological excitement. The energy impulses they transmit have abnormal frequencies. If there are damaged tissues in other areas of the body, this leads to resonance, followed by inflammation and catabolism. The cells are then unable to receive normal command impulses and to respond to them. They are no longer sensitive to normal neural stimulus.

Ferdinand Huneke, the founder of neural therapy, showed that the distant symptoms caused by a primary focus may be removed almost instantly by the injection of a local anaesthetic. The discovery came about, as so many important discoveries do, by chance. One day in 1929, his sister visited his office in Düsseldorf, Germany, complaining of an acute migraine and local pains in the arm. Meaning to ease temporarily the pain in the arm, Huneke injected it with a small dose of the fast-acting local anaesthetic, Novocain. By mistake, he injected it directly into a vein. Almost immediately, his sister's migraine disappeared. It was the beginning of neural therapy.

As we have seen, the cells within a focus are depolarised. By injecting a focus, or the area nearby, with a local anaesthetic such as Novocain, they are repolarised—and the distant symptoms induced by this focus will disappear; the local humoral and cellular milieu of the focal disturbance will gradually be normalised; necroses and infiltrations will be reduced. If there is more than one focus, causing distant effects therefore in many areas, only the relevant distant effects for the focus that has been anaesthetised will disappear.

Naturally such neural treatment of the distant effects must always be accompanied by surgical or other treatment of their cause, the primary focus.

Oxygen-ozone therapy has long been used in Germany and elsewhere for treating a variety of chronic diseases. Since the 1960s it has been increasingly used, with equal success, for treating cancer.

Normal molecular oxygen is a stable element which does not break down without a catalyst. On the other hand ozone has a distinct tendency to disintegrate into molecular oxygen and ionised (atomic) oxygen, which is a biologically active agent. In this form it is either injected into a patient intravenously, subcutaneously, or administered through the rectum.

After application the ozone reacts in four ways in the organism:

1. It increases bactericidal and virocidal activity.
2. It activates the aerobic metabolism in normal and malignant cells while inactivating the anaerobic metabolism.
3. It produces lipoid hydroperoxydes when combined with vitamin F. These are extremely effective aerobic catalysts with an effect similar to that of aerobic enzymes.
4. It reacts with and causes the elimination of oxidation-resistant toxic substances, especially such agents as the insecticides, pesticides, and other fat-soluble substances generally deposited in the connective tissue and other systems of the mesenchyme. Unless they are removed the mesenchymal activities are extensively blocked.

Therapeutically, ozone is administered twice a week. Each patient should initially receive a dose of 20 millilitres. This is regularly increased by degrees of 5 millilitres until the optimal dosage of 30 millilitres is reached. The important thing is continuity in treatment and a careful monitoring of results.

In cases where the tumour is on the skin or just below it, infusions of ozone may be directly injected into the lesion area, affording the maximum chances for immediate and beneficial results.

Haematogenic Oxydation Therapy, H.O.T., developed by the Swiss worker Wehrli, has been increasingly used since the early 1960s as part of modern medicine's arsenal against cancer.

Unlike many other treatments, H.O.T. is essentially simple, and has the added advantage of being painless. A quantity of blood, which, depending on the patient's state, can range from 100 to 200 hundred millilitres, is drawn off. Under suitable laboratory conditions, oxygen is then bubbled through it. This produces an effervescent effect and the foamed blood, previously usually blackish in colour, is now generally changed to a distinctive red. At this stage it is irradiated by ultra-violet rays for between five and ten minutes. Finally it is left to settle for up to an hour. Then it is returned to the patient by drip.

In treating blood in this manner, oxygen is transformed into ozone. The result is that the oxygenated blood derives the same benefits as it would from ozone therapy. The blood itself is sterilised, normalised, regenerated and reactivated. Defence cells regain their aggressive capacity. Returned to the host these cells can once more attack microbes and cancer-promoting viruses which are characterised by an anaerobic metabolism—making them unable to survive in the actively oxydised environment that H.O.T. creates. At the same time, malignant cells are attacked, alien and alienated proteins and other unwanted compounds in the blood are chemically altered during H.O.T., so that they can be recognised as such and eliminated.

H.O.T. is a regular weekly treatment which can go on for two or three months. There is no fixed time-scale; it depends on a number of factors, such as the condition of the patient at the onset of treatment, the progress and type of tumour. Needless to say, close clinical observation is necessary. If a patient is anaemic, blood from a donor must be used and treated in this manner before being drip-fed to the patient.

Hot-Ether-Therapy, developed by the German surgeon Tiegel, has still to gain wide acceptance even though clinical experience indicates it can destroy cancer cells. Heated to around 175°F., ether is inhaled. In this vaporised form it dissolves pathological lipids and their concomitant toxic compounds within the tissues, converting them into a transportable form. The lipoids can then be channelled out through the kidneys and intestines. Thus are the body's most dangerous ballast and waste materials excreted.

Many harmful toxins in the body combine with, or are bound to, the lipoid components of the blood and tissues: they are liposoluble. These toxins may be dangerous carcinogens, storing themselves in lipoids, especially within the lipoidal membranes of the cell. Attached to these membranes are hundreds of different enzyme molecules. There can be no doubt that if they are in any way damaged, for instance by the liposoluble toxins, normal cellular metabolism will be seriously affected.

Within malignant cells, the lipoidal membranes have themselves been converted into malignant lipoids, changed into malignolipin and similar compounds. These malignant membranes are highly vulnerable to liposoluble toxins. Consequently, in a chronically-ill body, there are large quantities of pathological lipoids present. Being inert, they are seldom detoxicated and eliminated; they remain lodged in storage mesenchymal cells until the vaporised ether dissolves them.

The actual treatment is simple. The patient is fitted with a mask that covers nose and mouth. From this mask, a flexible tube leads back to a heated chamber. Fresh air passes through this chamber and thus to the patient. Additionally, ether is dripped into the chamber—usually fifty drops a minute—and is instantly vaporised as it touches the hot casing. In this way the patient inhales a mixture of fresh air and ether vapour. The concentration of ether can of course be altered by increasing or decreasing the interval between the drops. Under the supervision of a doctor or nurse, the patient is encouraged to inhale slowly and steadily; medical supervision is required to control the flow rate of the gas, its temperature and to ensure the patient does not remove the face mask more often than necessary.

A dose of one-half gramme of hot ether per kilo of body weight is delivered. This is gradually increased until a maximum of one gramme per kilo of body weight is vaporised. The treatment then continues at this dosage for three to four weeks. Each session should last for as many minutes as one-half the number of kilos of body weight. For example, a patient weighing 80 kilos would inhale a maximum of 80 grammes of ether in 40 minutes.

Over the past twenty years I have increasingly seen the beneficial effects of this treatment in hundreds of cases, including the removal of depressive psychosis.

Auto-Hormone Therapy, passing ultra-short waves through the brain and its hormone-producing glands, can break the typical autonomic freeze of the cancer patient. Repeated at clinically indicated intervals, it can normalise the autonomic control functions and thereby eliminate one of the most important causal factors of the disease.

The autonomic, vegetative, centres of the brain, especially the thalamic and hypothalamic regions, respond to the irritative effect of the ultra-short waves by altering the body's metabolic reactions. There is an increase in hormone production. This, in addition to its immediate physiological result, will have a feedback effect within all the regulatory organs. Thus, this double-pronged attack not only initiates short-term normalisation of neuro-hormonic activity, but it also has a "training" effect whereby, in the course of time, the hormone-producing organs will begin again to spontaneously fulfil their biological tasks without the need for further ultra-short wave treatment.

Tumours which have hitherto shown themselves resistant to X-ray therapy can be made more susceptible by a preceding course of ultra-short waves: these will also allow for a reduction in the amount of X-rays needed, and this can only help to remove some of the unpleasant side-effects that so often accompany radiation.

Rehydration and a high fluid intake assist these treatments by eliminating the products of oncolysis and metabolic residues and improve liver and kidney function.

Pyretotherapy, the induction of high fever under clinical conditions, is an integral part of the whole-body concept of cancer treatment. Today its value is increasingly being recognised in Britain and the United States where a number of doctors have reported on the benefits accruing from it.

The idea that induced fever might be used to treat patients with a chronic disease like cancer is actually not new, nor is it claimed to be. The technique, once known as *malariatherapy or malarialisation*, from the idea of inducing malaria, has been used by Julius Vagner von Jauregg (1857–1940), for the treatment of syphilis and its rather gruesome aftermath, locomotor ataxia. Some 2,400 years ago, Hippocrates referred to the way in which many diseases—convulsions, epilepsy and "maniacal attacks"—could be controlled by concurrent malarial fever, one of the means of provoking the body into producing an *active* fever. Later, Parmenides wrote, somewhat optimistically: "Give me the means of producing a fever and I shall be able to cure all diseases".

The body's temperature is regulated by a "temperature centre" in the tuber cinereum of the midbrain. If microbial toxins circulating in the blood irritate this centre, a total change in the autonomous system occurs, causing extreme sympathicotonia. As a result, the body's metabolism is increased, its temperature rises, creating a "general febrile reaction", alerting all the defence mechanism of the body.

In such febrile conditions, active defence cells, neutrophilic granulocytes, are mobilised in the bone marrow and released into the blood. There is a marked increase in the number of leucocytes; the "active defence phase" has been reached which can be seen in the blood count. These defence cells produce bactericidal substances and also proteolytic and detoxicating enzymes. They are able to "swallow up" toxins, microbes and fragments of cells, storing them until they are dissolved in a process known as phagocytosis.

The production of specific antibodies, or "defence enzymes", by "immunocytes" (lymphocytes, lymph cells) is also greatly increased. Even a single feverish attack of a few hours' duration may, in some circumstances, cause antibody titres in the blood to increase ten times. In addition, febrile reactions stimulate the mobilisation and elimination of unwanted inert deposits in the mesenchymal stores. They clear toxicants remaining after acute and congenital infections, for instance congenital TB or syphilis. The elimination and regeneration of damaged tissue may be speeded up. Alkalosis is simultaneously converted into a relative acidosis, so that the internal environment of the body undergoes a fundamental change. In short, during general febrile reactions, the natural resistance and recuperative powers of the organism are brought to a high pitch.

Whole-body therapists know that the "delicate" child, the one who goes down with one paediatric infection after another, will, later in life, be less susceptible to chronic disease. And doctors believing in biological methods of treatment will always aim to promote and assist this most powerful curative reaction by, for instance, using hot mustard packs. These are particularly indicated when cutaneous eruptions "don't want to come out", when they "turn inwards", when the body's own febrile reaction is not powerful enough to overcome the infection without artificial stimulation.

Yet, contemporary medical thinking still does not generally regard heightened temperature as a curative reaction, but rather as something harmful to the body. Indeed, every attempt is usually made to suppress infections soon after they begin, with penicillin and other antibiotics. Nearly all of the drugs used nowadays against infectious and inflammatory diseases contain antibiotics or cortisone, substances which prevent inflammatory and contemporary feverish reactions.

If the organism is unable, or is not allowed, to develop an autonomic febrile reaction to rid itself completely of the toxins of infection, these have to be deposited in the storage cells of the mesenchyme. Residual toxicosis will result. And this will further reduce the remaining storage capacity, and simultaneously the ability of immunocompetent tissues to react. Finally, there may develop a mesenchymal "block" in parallel with a lowering of resistance, providing one of the major preconditions for the development of chronic diseases such as cancer.

It seems highly significant to me that many cancer patients have been previously "healthy" all their lives, their earlier medical record "blank". Usually they have not had any of the more serious febrile illnesses, and they have therefore not rid themselves of congenital and residual toxicosis.

M. von Ardenne, Lampert and others have shown that cancer cells are very sensitive to heat. At a temperature of around 105°F. the malignant cells in the body can be adversely damaged. On the other hand, healthy cells are not damaged until a temperature of 109.5°F. is reached. Fever and hyperthermia therefore not only improve the potency of defence, but also weaken cancer cells to such an extent that they can be destroyed more quickly by the defence mechanisms—while healthy cells go unharmed.

Lampert reported that inoculated tumours do not "take" if the host animals are given a hot bath before the tumour cells are injected. With experimental tumours, too, growth can thus be considerably slowed down; in certain cases, complete regression may occur.

A further benefit is that, if a patient is being treated by intermittent massive-dose chemotherapy, the drug dosage can be reduced by a third, sometimes even by a half, if it is administered at the peak of pyretotherapy. The curative effect is almost the same but there is a reduction in the harmful side-effects associated with chemotherapy.

The value of pyretotherapy is therefore established, in my view, beyond dispute, and the method has indeed proved its value in practice. It allows the internal milieu of a cancer patient to be improved, for blocked channels to be opened—including opening the all-important "filter" of the large intestine—and it improves resistance to tumour growth.

For these reasons, I utilise induced fever whenever possible. This may be done by inducing an *active* fever, for instance by the injection of a bacterial substance to which the body will react, or by the production of a *passive* fever—that is, when a febrile reaction is provoked artificially, usually from outside the body.

Active fever may be induced by injection of the drug Pyrifer, an ethical preparation. Made from coli bacteria specially treated, it irritates the fever control mechanism in the midbrain, and in about four hours, the body temperature is raised.

I generally induce passive fever by placing the patient inside a custom-built cylinder containing electrodes which emit ultra-short waves. Completely enclosed, the body is bombarded from head to toe with these waves, and literally within a few minutes, its temperature begins to rise. If the patient is able, and willing, to endure it—and here the doctor/patient relationship is extremely important—the temperature is kept at 105°F. for between one and one-and-a-half hours: the temperature at which cancer cells, but not normal cells, are damaged. Naturally, during this treatment the body loses potassium, and this must be balanced by a diet which is rich in potassium, for instance bananas, rice, or potatoes.

There are many other means of inducing passive fever, such as simply by giving the patient a hot bath and afterwards surrounding the body with hot water bottles and blankets. In this way the fever may be maintained for five or even six hours.

Passive fever treatment is usually repeated twice a week, sometimes for months, until the desired results are achieved. During this time, it is important that pyretotherapy is sympathetically but firmly administered, its value carefully explained, and whenever possible, the patients taught to regularly keep their own temperature chart.

I also recommend that pyretotherapy is continued as a follow-up treatment for some months further, on an outpatient basis, especially as by then the patients no longer fear the treatment, and in my experience take an active interest in it. Nevertheless, some family doctors refuse to give fever treatment because they still believe that an induced febrile reaction may be harmful.

That such attitudes exist today demonstrates how far localist beliefs can take us from perceiving the disease process as something involving the whole body. It is an unhappy example of why so many find themselves unable to treat chronic diseases, including cancer, in a successful, causal, way.

Substitution therapy includes all the measures aimed at restoring organic malfunction, by:

the substitutive stimulation of detoxicating and defensive systems, by liver and mesenchymal extracts etc.;
the regeneration of extremely stressed organs, by organ-specific RNA and DNA preparations;
the normalisation of metabolic malfunctions resulting from enzymatic defects, by regular application of specific drugs, as well as vitamins, minerals, etc.;
the administration of proteolytic enzymes to replace the missing non-specific dissolving activity.

Again, while the basic therapy regime may appear complicated, in practice it is not. It is also reproducible. Further, the more effective the general measures, the less there is a need for substitution.

The concurrent specific tumour therapy consists of surgery where possible, chemotherapy where indicated, radiotherapy where necessary. All these methods must always be combined with immunotherapy.

Active and *passive* immunisation, as well as immune stimulation, is effected with standard preparations.

All these specific measures can be optimised when integrated within the framework of the basic therapy. And an important part of that therapy is proper attention to foci.

8

Focus on Foci

THE "FOCUS" HAS BEEN DESCRIBED AS A CHRONIC, ABNORMAL, LOCAL change in the connective tissue, capable of producing the most varied distant effects beyond its immediate surroundings, and therefore in constant conflict with local and general defence (Pischinger and Kellner). By this definition, even a fully-healed scar may sometimes act as a focus, spreading disease to distant parts of the body. But the foci we shall now examine will be confined to those of the teeth and tonsils—in my view, the most lethal of all foci.

The emphasis I place on the removal of devitalised teeth and chronically-diseased tonsils is one of the better-known aspects of my work, but also one of the most criticised and misunderstood. I *do not*, for instance, recommend that healthy tonsils and teeth be removed from a healthy person. But I believe if they are diseased, they cause the body's natural resistance to be lowered, thus acting as an important contributory factor to tumour development. In these cases, I insist on their removal.

It is sometimes argued that to carry out such operations on seriously ill patients is unnecessarily cruel, even irrelevant. There are some unpleasant side-effects, but in my opinion, the benefits—which I will describe—more than make up for any temporary discomfort. It is further argued that in the cancer patient, as much lymphatic tissue as possible should be preserved, and that therefore tonsillectomy should not be carried out because even a diseased tonsil may retain some useful defence potential. I used to believe this was so. I do not any longer for reasons which will become evident.

The beneficial results of tonsillectomy with cancer patients were first brought to my attention in 1953, and by chance. A tonsillectomy was performed on an incurable cancer patient in my clinic who had severe rheumatic pains and a long history of tonsillar disease. The operation was done to relieve the woman's pain, but it was remarkably successful in other ways as well: general toxic symptoms disappeared, and, most important of all, her pathologically rapid pulse rate was reduced. Many cancer patients have a high pulse rate, reaching 140 and even 160, and this always leads to a poor prognosis, but in the case of this woman, it was almost normalised. Soon her tumour began to regress, and ultimately she recovered from her cancer.

This unexpected but welcome result encouraged me to arrange for tonsillectomies on two further patients with tonsillar ailments, who also had therapy-resistant cardiovascular disorders and toxic symptoms. In these cases as well, following surgery, cardiovascular and many other symptoms virtually disappeared. A positive "re-tuning" of natural defence and a certain inhibition of tumour growth was also observed. This improved situation naturally allowed more time for active immunotherapy to work.

These early successes encouraged me to persevere with tonsillectomies. Before making them virtually obligatory in my clinic, forty percent of those who died there did so from heart attacks. Afterwards the figure dropped to five percent. This, I contend, is incontrovertible proof that tonsillogenic toxins find their way into the bloodstream and eventually can cause, for instance, a fatal myocardial disease. This is one reason why more people die from heart disease than from any other.

In addition, my experience shows a direct connection between dental and tonsillar foci and many of the illnesses responsible for early debilitation and untimely invalidising.

It has long been generally accepted that head foci may give rise to almost all kinds of chronic, and certain acute diseases, such as—to mention a few—the manifold varieties of rheumatic and cardiovascular conditions. The removal of such foci is today a routine part in the conventional treatment of those diseases. However, the fact that head foci are also a contributory cause in the development of neoplasia, by lowering resistance, has received all too little acknowledgement.

The extent of the disease-provoking activity of a focus in distant parts of the body depends on whether the body is able to oppose the focus with its own defence mechanism. As long as the focal situation is kept under control by the local defence mechanism, no focus-induced remote effects will arise. On the other hand, distant effects will arise when the body's resistance has more or less broken down: control of head foci will then gradually collapse, and there will be a consequential gradual increase in generalised focogenic intoxication. This will cause an inevitable deterioration of the body's defence power with a con- comitant promotion of malignant growth.

Nearly everybody is confronted with dental problems at some time in their life, and even the most scrupulous dental care cannot guarantee dental health. Endogenous factors, such as prenatal damage to the embryonic dental tissue, as well as exogenous influences, such as malnutrition and toxins, must essentially be held responsible for the great number of dental diseases, be they a weak, susceptible gingiva, or gum; or teeth which are malpositioned, barrelled or impacted; or, worst of all, a disposition to decay.

Despite its porcelain-like surface, the crown enamel of the tooth is vulnerable to decay. Enamel defects develop especially in the grooves of the crown or on the adjacent surface of neighbouring teeth which are difficult to clean.

Decay is not painful so long as it is confined to this nerveless enamel layer. The onset of a toothache is the first noticeable sign that the decay has invaded the dentine body of the tooth which, unlike the enamel, does have nerves. If this decay is allowed to continue, sooner or later the dentine will be completely penetrated, and the pulp inside the tooth will then become inflamed.

As long as only the outer enamel and dentine are affected, the tooth can be preserved. But a tooth with an inflamed pulp can no longer be saved, and must be extracted without delay.

In an understandable desire to preserve as many teeth as possible, to maintain the masticatory apparatus and its functions, attempts are often made to save teeth which are in fact lost. There is a widespread conviction that this can be done without risk by the sterile evacuation of the pulp, and then refilling the cavity. For decades, the erroneous belief was held that, after such treatment, the tooth is an isolated, lifeless thing, no longer involved in any of the body's processes. This assumption was originally based on the premise that the pulp cavity had only one orifice to the apex of the root below, and by filling, this opening was sealed. However, the dentinal canal does not end in just one opening; instead, it resembles a tree with many branches which penetrate the tooth's body in all directions.

The finer details of the entire dental structure have been exhaustively studied by Austrian researchers. They have established that there is a lively metabolic interchange between the interior and exterior milieu of the tooth, and that this two-way process takes place along many thousands of hyperfine, capillary canals joining the pulp cavity to the exterior surface of the tooth.

Very careful conservation measures may possibly seal off the vertical central-medial-tube of the dentinal canal, but it will never reach the lateral "twigs" branching off from this tube. Nor can it ever close off the innumerable capillary canals. Some protein will always remain in these secondary spaces. If this protein becomes infected, toxic catabolic products will be produced, and conveyed into the organism.

It was established in 1960 by W. Meyer (Göttingen) that within devitalised teeth the dentinal canals and dental capillaries contain large microbial colonies. The toxins produced by these microbes in a tooth with a root filling can no longer be evacuated into the mouth, but must be drained away through the cross-connections and unsealed branches of the dentinal and capillary canals into the marrow of the jawbone. From there, they are conveyed to the tonsils, and thus the flow systems of the body. In fact, the conservation treatment may literally convert a tooth into a toxin producing "factory".

A devitalised tooth is no longer able to perceive and control inflammatory processes even when suppuration has invaded the surrounding bone spaces of the tooth's socket; it rarely gives warning signals, for instance through pain, and therefore there is nothing to induce the patient to have this dangerous toxic foci removed. It then may be left to develop its devastating effect on the organism for decades or even for a lifetime.

When the inflammation spreads to the marrow of the tooth socket, it can cause osteomyelitis. Its further course is determined by whether and for how long the local defence is able to keep the focal disturbance under control.

If the body's local resistance is intact, the inflammation is enclosed by a capsule of connective tissue known as the dental granuloma. This membranous cyst prevents its toxic contents from spreading into the organism. Radiographs of these teeth show granuloma cysts as more or less marked transparencies at the apex of the root. This type of tooth is called X-ray positive.

If the body's local resistance is weakened to such an extent that the inflammatory process cannot be encapsulated by the granuloma cyst, the toxins will be able to advance unhindered into the marrow spaces, the tonsils, and into the body. In this case, it is proof that—as stressed by Pischinger and Kellner—the organism has become largely incapable of reaction. Radiographs of these teeth as a rule show no transparencies, and are therefore called X-ray negative.

In my cancer patients, I have found that such non-encapsulated foci— that is those who show X-ray negative—were particularly common, as one would expect from people whose body resistance had been lowered.

Today there is general agreement that dental foci should be cleared away, and it has become usual to diagnose them by X-ray. Unfortunately, only some of the dental foci can be discovered by this means. Encapsulated foci can be recognised only if large enough, and if not concealed by the tooth's shadow. And definite X-ray signs are much rarer in non-encapsulated osteomyelitic processes. It is therefore the most dangerous of all dental foci which most frequently prove X-ray negative. Even with X-ray positive dental film, only those foci can be recognised which happen to be situated outside shadows. Since X-ray negative foci often escape treatment—and they are the ones the body has failed to resist effectively—they can continue to develop their destructive effects unhindered.

My clinical experience has produced evidence of a causal connection between foci and tumour development, and in this respect, the results obtained with the aid of an infra-red test are especially significant.

Any inflammatory disease focus creates on its corresponding skin surface a pathological increase of infra-red emission; the higher the activity of the focus, the more pronounced it is. Using an infra-red-sensitive instrument (Schwamm's infra-red toposcope), the intensity of this emission can be continuously monitored and measured. Observation showed a close interrelation between the infra-red emission of head foci and that of the neoplasial region. That is, after treatment, a decrease in the infra-red activity of dental foci was as a rule accompanied by a decrease in infra-red emission over the tumour areas.

From this it is clear that the advisable treatment for devitalised teeth is extraction.

But even this is not always enough. My experience has further shown that also living teeth may sometimes be so damaged that their pathogenic potential almost equals that of devitalised teeth. For instance, latent chronic pulpitis may arise in a tooth that appears outwardly healthy, thus having a focal effect.

The diagnosis and treatment of dental foci remains generally unsatisfactory. A survey conducted at my clinic found that, on admission, ninety-eight percent of the adult cancer patients had between two and ten dead teeth, each one a dangerous toxin producing "factory". Very often we are confronted with X-ray negative dead teeth, root remnants, and residual ostitis which had not been diagnosed and therefore had not been removed.

Only total, thorough dental treatment will really succeed in giving the body's defence a chance. In addition to X-ray diagnosis, it is therefore necessary to use other diagnostic aids, such as infra-red techniques, tests, to estimate tooth vitality and periosteal resistance, and other electrometric methods.

The diagnosis of foci in teeth has been greatly improved by electro-acupuncture. It is now possible to differentiate foci not only with regard to their type and position, but also to their virulence and pathogenic efficacy. The result of focus treatment can consequently be observed and improved, before, during, and after dentistry, to an extent never known before (Kramer).

If total treatment is to be performed, it is necessary to remove not only any devitalised teeth but also any hidden dental foci remaining in the jaw.

Further, total removal of devitalised teeth and their roots must not be the end of the dentist's activities. Each alveolus—the tooth's socket in the jaw—should be radically cleared down to the healthy bone. In that way the development of a residual ostitis or of a cystoma may be prevented. It is not only the tooth which may be a focus, but the adjacent tooth-fixing apparatus as well.

There are four different ways by which dental foci—and indeed all foci—can affect the organism and contribute to the development of secondary damages:

1. The "neural" way of affecting the organism.

When a focus develops anywhere in the transit tissues, the mesenchyme, the process is centripetally projected from the terminal neural organs around the irritated area, along the neural ducts, up to the corresponding control cells within the central nervous system. The irritation originating from a focus can, under certain conditions, trigger off the mechanism of a neural dystrophy—a slow degeneration—which may show itself in localised effects in other areas, but also in a generalised dystrophic disturbance.

In the 1950s it was shown that these manifestations are based on depolarising processes in the affected neural cells, and in the corresponding tissues of the body's periphery (Fleckenstein and Ernsthausen). By elimination of the focus, the affected tissues may be repolarised. The most striking example of this repolarisation is called "second-phenomenon".

Ferdinand Huneke, the founder of neural therapy whose remarkable contribution in this regard we shall look at in detail later, discovered over forty years ago that injection of a local anaesthetic near a primary focus may immediately remove any symptoms of distant disease induced by the focus. This effect—the second-phenomenon—usually takes place only a few seconds after the anaesthetic injection, and lasts for hours, days, or even for a lifetime. Naturally the improvement occurs only in those regions influenced by the injected focus. Nevertheless, the measure has therefore a remarkable diagnostic value as well.

Since neural therapy only neutralises the neural effect of a focus, the focus itself must, of course, be removed after such treatment, in order to eliminate its latent toxic or allergenetic action. Conversely, any focal surgery must be followed by desensitising and neural-therapeutic measures.

The only exceptions to this rule are, for instance, featureless scars or other spots with no inflammatory change which produce only neural distant effects without at the same time causing any toxic, microbial, or allergic secondary phenomena.

2. The "toxic way" of affecting the organism.

The toxic activity of odontogenic foci is probably far more perilous for the organism than their neural effects. The mechanism of this distant toxic activity, as well as the characteristics of the toxic compounds involved, have been largely ascertained.

Odontogenic compounds are the gangrenous contents of an inflamed pulp cavity and its adjoining spaces. It consists of detritus and decaying, formerly vital substrates which have been necrobiotically altered—

commonly found in tissues destroyed by inflammation, liquefaction and microbial putrefaction. Thus there can be little doubt that they are genuine necrogenous toxins, including for instance autologous proteinic and higher-molecular proteinogenous compounds. Later there will be produced numerous low-molecular fission products resulting from enzyme cleavage and other biogenic conversions.

The identity and chemical structure of certain of the biogenic amines were mainly clarified in the 1950s by Schug-Koesters, Hiller, Gaebelein and others of the University of Munich. Following similar findings in America, the metabolic and exchange processes in solid dental structures were further investigated by the German researcher Spreter von Kreudenstein. He showed that drugs injected intravenously were, four to five hours later, discernible within the intradental capillary ducts or even devitalised teeth, and in a concentration only slightly lower than in the blood.

That endodental exchange may also take place in the opposite direction has been reported by Bartelstone (USA) and Djerassi (Bulgaria). If radio-iodine, I–131, is deposited in an evacuated pulp cavity which is then sealed off with a filling, the iodine will appear in the thyroid some twenty hours later, as can be demonstrated by taking a scintograph of the thyroid region. Similarly, dyes can be washed out of a sealed pulp cavity.

All these findings prove conclusively that within solid dental structures, there may proceed an unimpeded substantial interchange in either direction. Consequently, odontogenic toxins, wherever they may have been produced, are able to diffuse and circulate within the organism.

The pathogenic significance of these "endotoxins" has been investigated by the German study group of Eger-Miehlke. They examined the changes in healthy experimental animals after injection of accurately defined, minimal quantities of the endotoxins from an odontogenous granuloma.

A single injection of a minimal dose seemed to develop a defence-activating effect. But after repeated injections, there was severe liver damage, and the animals died within weeks. Apart from the fatal liver damage, inflammatory and degenerative changes were found in all other organs, especially in the joints, muscles, and blood vessels.

These results brought clear experimental proof for the first time that focogenic toxins act as causal agents for severe diseases in animals corresponding to similar chronic conditions in man.

The most dangerous of all odontogenous toxins are undoubtedly the thio-ethers, for instance dimethylsulfide. In a series of tests performed at my clinic, it was observed that patients with odontogenous and tonsillar foci had a heightened level of dimethylsulfide in their blood. After intensive treatment of the foci, this level returned to normal in just a few days.

Thio-ethers are closely related, both in their structure and their effect, to mustard gas and other poison gases used in the First World War. The extreme toxicity of the poison gases and thio-ethers can be attributed to the following properties:

1. They are weakly basic, therefore "electro-negative", and thus they are deposited particularly in "electro-positive" cells such as those of the transit tissues as well as those of the defensive tissues.
2. They are soluble in the lipids, and therefore have a pronounced tendency to enrich themselves in the lipoid-containing cellular structures, especially in mitochondria.
3. These subcellular organelles, attached to their lipoid membranes, contain the enzymatic structures responsible for the maintenance of aerobic metabolism—a precondition for full functioning power in all the body's cells and tissues. If these indispensable units are damaged, the most serious consequences will follow. Because they are the most vulnerable cellular organelles, mitochondria are a favourite and almost exclusive target for thio-ethers.

The action of thio-ethers is effected in three main ways:

a) Since thio-ethers tend to combine with electro-positive metal ions and many bio-elements which act as co-effectors or activators of numerous enzymes of absolutely vital importance, and as our present-day average diet is deficient in essential substrates such as vitamins and bio-metals, this deficiency is enhanced. Much of the daily intake of bio-metals, usually deposited in the fluids of a focally affected organism, will be made permanently ineffective; the more foci, the greater will become the deficiency.
b) Thio-ethers are "partial" antigens, haptens, and thus they also tend to combine with the normal proteins in the body, "denaturising" them. Such denatured proteins become "non-self" agents which the body must deal with as such. The production of antibodies adapted to the situation will be provoked, and they will home in on

the target antigens wherever they are. The process of "auto-aggression" will be set in motion: self-destruction of agents alien to the organism. Extensive structural cellular damage will result, increasing with age.

c) The famous biologist, Otto Warburg, twice winner of the Nobel Prize, has shown that aerobically-blocked cells—as caused by thio-ethers—will increase their anaerobic metabolism in an attempt to maintain their vigour. In doing so, they acquire the characteristics of malignant cells. Therefore, chemical agents capable of inactivating the aerobic process while increasing the anaerobic process are usually classed as carcinogenous compounds.

Druckrey (Heidelberg) found *inter alia* that transformation of a normal cell into a malignant cell requires a certain quantity of a carcinogen —the carcinogenic minimum dose. It does not matter whether this quantity is supplied in a single dose or in a number of smaller doses, because the toxic effects of each dose are stored, and accumulate without loss. The carcinogens held primarily responsible for the development of spontaneous cancer in man are those:

which inhibit the aerobiosis even in minimal quantities without at the same time immediately destroying the cell, and,

which are constantly present in the organism in this minimal concentration of either endogenous or exogenous origin; they can therefore accumulate during the normal life expectancy gradually and unnoticeably until the total quantity necessary for malignisation is reached.

There is hardly a carcinogen which so completely fulfils these conditions as do thio-ethers. Incessantly, from the moment the pulp is removed, hour by hour, year by year, minimal amounts of these most virulent of all the odontogenous toxins will be released into the circulation—minimal doses, but nevertheless sufficient to more or less totally paralyse the aerobic action of the cell.

The nervous system is thus doubly affected by focal intoxication. Firstly, by the increasing destruction of the neural ducts which mediate between the control centres and the peripheral areas, thus sometimes initiating neurogenic dystrophy. And secondly, by the immediate intoxication of neural cells caused by the toxins spreading through the liquid vehicles of the flow systems, such as the blood and lymph.

The more mitochondria a cell contains, the more it will be damaged by the enzyme-inhibiting effect of thio-ether compounds. Therefore it is the vital organs—the liver, nervous system, endocrine glands, heart, and reticuloendothelial system—whose cells may consist of up to one-fifth of mitochondria, that are primarily affected. Apart from disturbing regulatory control, odontogenous toxins will also cause additional damage almost throughout the body. Naturally, the higher the blood-level of focogenous toxins, the more severe will be their effect.

The close interlacing of the lymphatic and endocrine systems in the head, make it unavoidable that brain cells are more intensively toxified by the circulating focogenous agents and may suffer particularly heavy damage. The lymph ducts of the head region join Waldeyer's tonsillar ring where detoxification takes place. There, inflammatory swellings inevitably cause a lymphatic congestion. All the toxic sewage of head foci are channelled into Waldeyer's tonsillar ring, and if there is such congestion, waste fluids will be pressed through the porous base of the skull into the lymphatic spaces of the brain. Toxogenous changes, especially within autonomic nuclei, are regularly found in cancer patients, as verified in the 1930s by Muehlmann (USSR), and they may be a consequence of a life-long inhibition of cerebral aerobiosis due to focogenous intoxication.

The cerebral damage (diencephalosis) and the subsequent loss of vitality in cancer patients is accompanied by a number of other symptoms. The emission of hypothalamic energy impulses, recordable by a Voll's electro-acupuncture device, are reduced in patients with focal disease. The autonomic vigour is relaxed, creating "regulation rigidity": carcinomas tend to parasympathicotonic derailment; in sarcomas and systemic diseases, as a rule the opposite is found—sympathicotonic derailment (Regelsberger, Gratzl-Martin, Rilling et al). The diurnal, circadian regulation of the acid-base balance is lost (Sander). At the same time, there will exist a distinct inhibition of other diurnal control functions, for instance of blood sugar, cholesterol, and mineral metabolism, and many other metabolic parameters are greatly restricted (Hinsberg).

The lack of vigour and control efficiency is not, of course, without effect on the patient's psychic condition. Vegetative disorder is therefore generally accompanied by neurasthenic dystonia—characterised by the diminishing vitality and autonomic instability.

3. The "allergic" way of affecting the organism.

The toxic effects of thio-ethers overlap those caused by higher-molecular odontogenous toxins, as already described.

Antibodies are formed to fight these substances, eventually leading to the destructive processes in toxified cells. Since the organ-destroying antibodies or defence enzymes are excreted by the kidneys, they can be diagnosed in the urine by the Abderhalden test. In this way we can precisely deduce, in most cases, which organs have suffered secondary damage (Abderhalden, Dyckerhoff et al).

The extent of secondary lesions can also be demonstrated indirectly by vaccine treatment. Using desensitising vaccines made from foco-genous agents, reactions are caused in regions affected by distant focal effects which may become evident in regional as well as general symptoms.

It is thus clear that the development of cancer disease is, in more ways than one, closely linked with focal events.

4. The "bacterial" way of affecting the organism.

Bacterial dissemination from primary dental foci as a rule takes place with barely perceptible symptoms, and may be followed by the formation of "secondary foci" in other regions. These include, inter alia, foci in the paranasal sinuses, gall-bladder, appendix, prostate, and renal pelvis.

Above all, bacterial dissemination tends to produce microfoci or microthrombi in veins, and they in turn have a tendency to thrombosis or thrombophlebitis, possibly with concomitant embolism.

Thrombophlebitis and thrombosis, so common in cancer patients, and generally regarded as resulting from disordered metabolism, are due not only to the dyscrasia of those patients, but also to the manifold effects of dental foci.

Shakow (Moscow), in collaboration with several clinics, has carried out an interesting investigation involving more than 1200 young pupils at a boarding school. Over a period of six years, it was seen that students with devitalised teeth had three times as many illnesses as those with healthy dentition. By removing devitalised teeth in these young patients, up to eighty percent of their illnesses were cured.

We have now seen how decisively the entire organism is affected by dental foci not properly treated, and what catastrophic results destruction of the pulp may entail. Dentists must, therefore, bear in mind that there is no root treatment which does not inevitably produce foci.

The dentist's task is only secondarily cosmetic; primarily it must be preventive and curative. The over-riding consideration must not be conservation of the tooth but preservation of its vitality. If this is impossible, even the most beautiful crown must not delude us that the lifeless tooth beneath is anything other than a "corpse in a golden coffin", whose decomposition toxins slowly but surely are destroying the organism (Bircher-Benner).

Other foci in the jaw, for instance ostitis, cysts, foreign bodies, gingivitis, and malposition of teeth may also develop focal effects. It goes without saying that these foci and centres of irritation must be removed.

The dentist should always remember that he has a vital role to prevent the development of chronic illness and, most important of all, to decisively reduce the hazard of cancer.

Now let us turn to tonsillar foci.

Chronically inflamed tonsils are primary head foci which sometimes have an even more damaging effect on the organism as a whole than dental foci. They can participate in the development of chronic illness, including cancer, by the four ways already described for dental foci: by neural, toxic, allergic, and bacterial means. There are also similar connections between the development of cancer and tonsillar foci as there are between cancer and dental foci. For instance, after removing the tonsils, there is a decrease of infra-red radiation over the tumour, and sometimes even a shrinking of the tumour.

The three tonsils in man, that is, the naso-pharyngeal tonsil, or adenoid, and the two tonsils proper, the palatine tonsils in the pockets between the anterior and posterior palatine arches in the back region of the mouth, together with other seemingly insignificant lymphoepithelial organs, form Waldeyer's tonsillar ring.

The tonsils are excretion organs by which the lymphocytes, microbes, toxin-laden lymph, and other matter, are discharged (Roeder). Even in healthy people, the tonsils may contain plugs—sometimes wrongly described as pus—which consist mainly of fatty acids, cholesterol, and other slag substances clearly characterising them as excretion. The pale-coloured plugs form in the shallow depressions on the tonsils' surface—the tonsillar crypts—and are expelled into the oral cavity and swallowed. The excretions of the tonsils may also contain dental toxins.

The tonsillar crypts have been described as the places where the physiologically obligatory bacterial flora are hatched. This flora colonises the mucous membranes of the nose and throat and the other air passages. The tonsils also produce antibodies, and undesirable microbes and their toxins are rendered harmless. Thus they have an immunising or detoxicating purpose and must be regarded as a functional analogue of the lymph organs of the intestinal mucous membrane, and, like the latter, as an important part of the body's defence system.

Healthy tonsils have a pale, pink, surface, and are normally almond or bean-sized. Their size and reaction capacity are determined not only by functional demands and loads, but also to some extent by each individual's inherited constitution. With an inherited disposition to lymphatic diathesis, due mainly to heavy hereditary infection, there is regularly found a congenital enlargement or hyperplasia of the tonsils. This is always accompanied by an increased disposition to inflammatory reactions. Inflammatory reactions are also caused by their physiological function. A normally subliminal, and therefore symptomless tonsillitis, thus belongs to the "normal bodily state of man" (Luescher).

Whenever large quantities of toxic and waste substances have to be excreted, the blood perfusion and inflammatory activity of the tonsils will increase. This state is often accompanied by painful swelling and reddening of the tonsils, and is described, depending on its subsequent course, as acute, sub-acute, or if occurring repeatedly, chronic tonsillitis.

I shall now concentrate on chronic, and especially on degenerative tonsillitis, because, under certain conditions, dangerous focal processes develop from it which are of causal importance for the origin of all chronic illnesses, including cancer.

Although each case of chronic tonsillitis is due to the same mechanism, it is possible to distinguish between three different groups.

The first group includes those chronic tonsillitis cases which arise in healthy tonsillar tissues capable of response, following frequent attacks of acute tonsillitis, or angina; they have been called upon to repeatedly react to infective irritation, and to excrete toxins. Each new attack leads to an increase in volume, perfusion, and activity. They are then in a high state of readiness for defence. But if such inflammations occur with increasing frequency, the tonsils gradually lose their reaction capacity and defensive power, and atrophy. Too much has been asked of them.

The second group includes those tonsillar foci which develop under certain conditions from congenitally enlarged or hyperplastic tonsils. This kind of hyperplasia can be so extensive that the fauces are completely obstructed. Unfortunately it is still common practice to reduce their size by partially lopping off these hyperplastic tonsils. The tonsils are thereby deprived of the shallow depressions—the crypts—so indispensable to their purpose; the excretory function cannot take place without an intact surface with open crypts. After a tonsillotomy lopping-off operation, the remaining crypts are always narrowed or closed by scar tissue, the substances to be excreted are cut off from their air supply (Voss), and are therefore un-aerobically decomposed with the formation of toxic decomposition products. It follows that lopping-off should not be performed. These tonsils should be totally removed, even if they are not yet causing any recognisable distant effects.

The third group of tonsillar foci, in cancer patients the most common, comprises the seemingly healthy, but small, congenitally under-developed and functionally deficient tonsils. A history of tonsillar symptoms is usually absent in these patients. Their tonsils are "un-remarkable", but firmly fused with their base, and cannot easily be dislodged.

What these three main groups of chronic tonsillitis have in common is a focal-toxigenic effect progressively increasing with age, and a tendency sooner or later to atrophy. This process will be accelerated if there is an additional and continuous passive exposure to odontogenous toxins.

The close connection between teeth and tonsils was proven when it was observed that Indian ink injected into a sealed dental cavity appeared as spots on the tonsillar surface in about twenty to thirty minutes. These experiments showed that pathogenic substances from the jaw region, including toxins from devitalised teeth, are conducted to the lymphatic tonsillar ring, there to be detoxicated and excreted. Besides their "natural" physiological load, the tonsils are thus additionally exposed to continuous attack by odontogenous toxins provoked by the devitalisation of teeth.

We have already seen how dangerous these dental toxins are. It is inevitable that they eventually have a severe effect on the active lymph-oepithelial tonsillar tissue. So long as the cells destroyed by dental toxins can be regeneratively replaced, the functional capacity of the tonsils will not be seriously impaired. But if the destroyed lymphoepi-thelial tissue is increasingly replaced by inactive scar tissue—by tissue unable to execute its defence function—the excretion, detoxication, and defence capacity of the tonsils will progressively diminish and eventually be extinguished.

With the loss of reactive lymphatic tissue, the tonsils lose their ability to give warning signs by inflammation; they no longer offer this usual signal for trouble. According to Kellner, this lack of symptoms signifies a definite inability to continue to further reaction. In such tonsils, the attacking toxins are no longer excreted; on the contrary, they are channelled into the organism via the vascular system.

It goes without saying that this development will take place far more quickly when less lymphoepithelial tissue is still present. In congenital tonsillar deficiency, there is, *a priori*, so little active tissue that its complete destruction can in certain cases be accomplished in a relatively short time. Normally developed, or hyperplastic tonsils if not lopped off, will withstand the dental infection considerably longer. But they too will sooner or later succumb.

The final stage of all three forms of chronic tonsillitis is therefore "atrophically degenerating tonsillitis". On medical examination, the findings here are small, atrophic tonsils which show no sign of inflam-mation but, unlike healthy tonsils, they cannot be dislodged by the surgeon's spatula. When removing them, they have to be dissected from their bed, so firmly fused are they to the surrounding tissue. Whereas with healthy tonsils the colour of the anterior palatine arch does not differ from that of the oral mucous membrane, in atrophically degen-erating tonsillitis there is a bluish discoloration of the palatine arch. The uvula is mostly gelatinously thickened. The tonsils themselves, however, may still appear externally healthy.

Even normal-sized or enlarged tonsils may already have extensive degenerative changes and consist mainly of hardened scar tissue which of course is unable to neutralise toxins. There then follows the forma-tion of usually quite latent and painless chronic tonsillar and retro-tonsillar abscesses. Here we find the highly pathogenic beta-haemolytic streptococci of Group A—responsible for many chronic illnesses, and whose toxins spread through the organism and contribute to the

development of secondary lesions, of resistance deficiency, and of the
tumour milieu.

Apart from the directly allergenic and toxinic activity of these
products, continuous toxic attack always leads to an alteration of the
tonsillar (lymphoid) cells. Their proteinic structure is so altered that the
organism is induced to form antibodies against these, its own, cells
which have become foreign to it, antibodies which finally turn against
healthy lymphocytes as well, and thus considerably weaken the
lymphatic defence system of the whole organism.

With the decline of the active tonsillar tissue, its biological power is
also exhausted. Active detoxication, toxicopexis, and excretion of toxic
substances and wastes through the tonsils is no longer possible. In the
tonsillar crypts, the physiologically essential symbionts are no longer
hatched. Instead, dangerous pathogenic organisms are able to spread
through the body because the immuno-activity of the tonsillar barrier
is lost with the destruction of the lymphoepithelial tissue.

When the dental toxins are no longer neutralised and excreted, they
will infiltrate even the last remnants of functioning tonsillar tissue and
cause them to die. This creates high- and low-molecular necrotoxins
which, as we have already seen, are similar or identical to odontogenous
toxins. Toxin formation is inevitably increased.

All these toxins, no longer inactivated in the tonsillar ring or excreted,
have to be conducted to other "vents" by way of the blood circulation.
Toxinaemia and secondary lesions are increased, and the humoral
milieu and the body's resistance deteriorates further. The process has
become a deadly vicious circle.

Since degenerated and chronically inflamed tonsils are such dangerous
toxogenic foci, like dead teeth and other dental foci, they must be
removed. With previously lopped tonsils, there is also a clear case for
tonsillectomy.

The focogenous toxicopathy caused by necrotic-atrophic tonsillitis is
of course far more dangerous than the toxi-infectious effect of a hyper-
reactive tonsillitis in childhood. And if the need for tonsillectomy is
accepted in children, in cases of rheumatism and other comparatively
harmless diseases, should it not be obeyed all the more urgently in
tumour disease, especially as a causal connection between focal and
tumour events can no longer be denied?

During more than twenty-five years of clinical experience, I have
found that painful, enlarged tonsils and other symptoms of chronic

tonsillitis were evident in less than one-third of my cancer patients. This suggested to me early on that the others might have silent tonsillar foci in the form of atrophically-degenerating tonsils. In these patients with subjectively quite unremarkable, small, featureless tonsils, I examined their case histories, and searched for silent tonsillar foci with the aid of the infra-red toposcope, the electrodermatometer, and other methods. These observations showed that, although most of them had never suffered from tonsillitis, there were clear findings of a tonsillo-genic focal toxicosis. Whenever this was compatible with the condition of the patient tonsillectomy was performed.

The findings in these healthy-looking tonsils were incomparably more serious than even those in the obviously diseased tonsils removed in usual ear-nose-and-throat practice. The tonsillar capsule always proved to show callous thickening, and was so firmly adherent that the tonsils could only be dissected out. In about five percent of the patients there were fairly large peritonsillary or retrotonsillary abscesses which had caused no symptoms. Far more frequently there were several abscesses as well as cysts often the size of cherries, full of liquid or condensed pus. The tonsillar tissue was spongy, slushy, and had a putrid smell. Histological examination of these tonsils always showed severe degenerative changes, and in the majority of cases, a complete atrophy of lymphoepithelial tissue.

All these "featureless", clinically unremarkable, small tonsils proved without exception to be foci of the most dangerous kind which, like the silent dental foci, had probably been present and unrecognised for years or even decades.

These pronounced positive effects of tonsillectomy make it manda-tory to always follow dentistry with treatment of the tonsils. In every tonsillectomy performed in my clinic subsequently, we found through biopsy severe or very severe destructive tonsillar processes with more or less virulent tonsillogenic focal toxicosis.

The flourishing of patients after tonsillectomy is impressive and has been demonstrated to my clinical satisfaction again and again.

Toxins constantly circulating in the blood in degenerative tonsillitis cause a permanent spasm of the blood capillaries, seen outwardly in the poorly perfused, pallid skin of many cancer patients. After tonsillectomy and the consequent elimination of the toxins and their neural effect, there was frequently an immediate improvement of the circulation and a simultaneous improvement in the general condition of the organism.

As already mentioned, before I began paying special attention to the tonsils, I lost many incurable patients, *not* as a result of cancer, but through acute cardiocirculatory failure. After introducing tonsillectomy, such deaths became much rarer.

Toxic circulatory death, however, is only one of the many dangers constantly threatening the life of the chronically sick. Phlebitis, thrombosis, embolism, pneumonia, pleurisy, and cystitis all too often complicate the course of treatment. In my experience, these, too, became noticeably rarer with the introduction of routine tonsillectomy.

Another observation, one I believe very important for cancer treatment, is that often following tonsillectomy, in a large proportion of patients, I have found that the tongue, not coated before the tonsillectomy, later has a marked yellowish, brownish, or blackish coating. Experience shows that the canalising activity of the intestinal mucous membranes is indicated by the surface condition or coating of the tongue; a change in this coating suggests that a previously blocked "gut filter" has been opened, leading to the conclusion that tonsillar foci also disturb the detoxicating and excretory activity of the gut. Restitution of this function is of crucial importance in the treatment of cancer because the largest proportion of the necrogenous toxins which develop during tumour solution is excreted by this route.

The widespread opinion that degeneratively destroyed tonsils may still be of importance for cancer patients as detoxicating and excretory organs and must therefore be preserved at all cost has, in my experience, been quite clearly refuted. Anyone, having seen the degenerative destruction in the tonsillar tissue of cancer patients, will be convinced that, on the contrary, these tonsils have contributed in potentiating the virulence of the tumour milieu and the defence deficiency.

Tonsillectomy must be followed by desensitisation with vaccines obtained from dental and tonsillar foci. Neural treatment of the tonsillar bed concludes this treatment.

The increased tendency towards thrombosis in cancer patients has been reported by many clinicians. It can be assumed there is a causal connection between the two diseases. My experience is that this tendency is reduced by treatment of the head foci. I have treated cancer patients who were being given anticoagulants permanently because of their thrombosis; after treatment of the head foci, as a rule, they were able to discontinue these drugs.

In some cancer patients there is a secondary finding of therapy-resistant hypertension. Here too, following treatment of the head foci, the blood pressure generally returns to normal.

The growth of the tumour itself is very often distinctly slowed down by focus treatment. Now and then tumour development stops altogether, and sometimes even regresses. The head foci therefore seem not only to contribute to the development of secondary lesions, to the origin of cancer disease, but also to exert a direct influence on tumour growth by stimulating it. Many tumours seem to respond to immunotherapy only when foci have been removed. The subsequent improvement in the body's defences clearly shows itself in the response to immunising vaccines.

Nevertheless, my own unhappy experience shows that with cancer patients, foci treatment has generally been left to a very late stage. In the vast majority of the patients I have treated, it was quite clear that foci treatment should have been carried out years before—and certainly long before the manifestation of the tumours.

That this was not done is a sad reminder that far too many doctors and dentists fail to recognise a fundamental truism: untreated foci can be linked to the development of cancer.

There are also other facets of our every day life-style that indirectly play their part in how the disease can progress.

9

Eat Well to Get Well

ALL CHRONIC DISEASES, INCLUDING CANCER, ARE TO A CERTAIN EXTENT
due to faulty nutrition. Therefore, a proper diet should have a positive
effect on chronic conditions. A well thought-out, biologically adequate
regime is an essential precondition for successful treatment.

Before examining the ingredients necessary for such a diet, let
us look at historical evolution of nutritional science.

The first real discoveries concerning the chemical composition of
food date from 1840. It was found that all food consists of three
basic organic substances: protein, fat, and carbohydrates. All other
constituents were at that time classified as "ash". A diet was thought to
be entirely adequate if the daily intake per kilogramme of body weight
was 1 gramme of protein, 1 gramme of fat, and 6 grams of carbohydrates. In fact this is much less than the body requires.

In 1875, Falk, Hofmann, and Forster defined the food requirements
in animals. They found that in addition to protein, fat, and carbohydrates, the ingredients of the "ash" were also essential for maintenance of life.

In 1881, Lunin came to the conclusion that Man's food must also
contain other vital elements of unknown structure, and in 1895/6,
Eijckmann finally succeeded in isolating the first of these substances—
the "beriberi preventive" factor—later known as B_1. In subsequent
years, about forty more "preventives" were found, and in 1929,
Funk suggested they should be called vitamins. Diseases caused by

inadequate intake of these nutritional factors were thus termed vitamin-deficient.

From 1923 onwards, Kollath carried out animal experiments to try to establish whether life and health could be supported using only the trace minerals and organic compounds which had so far been discovered. It became evident that apart from known vitamins and bio-elements, food must contain other elements if full health was to be maintained. The first of these are now known to be a number of active agents of the vitamin B group, the "auxons"—so-called because they stimulate growth and regeneration; the second are vital proteins in the form of fresh plant or animal food.

If the diet does not contain these auxons and vital proteins in sufficient quantity, a state of "semi-health" or mesotrophy develops, recognisable by the following symptoms and signs:

1. Inhibition of growth, defective regeneration
2. Dental and skeletal decay
3. Atrophy and depletion of ganglion cells, neural dys-function, autonomic and psycho-physiological disorders
4. Inhibition of hormonal function, particularly affecting the pituitary and adrenals, inadequate resistance to stress
5. Atrophy of the mesenchyme
6. Reduction of antibody formation and thus lowered resistance, and susceptibility to infections
7. Degeneration of the physiological obligatory intestinal flora, chronic constipation
8. Predisposition towards all forms of chronic disease, including cancer
9. Premature ageing
10. Reduced life-expectancy.

This catalogue shows a striking similarity to the damage sustained by Man through our present-day eating habits.

Indeed, analysis has shown that today's average diet contains very few auxons and live protein, certainly not enough to cover the body's minimum requirements. Our average diet must therefore be accurately described as a "mesotrophic diet".

Few details are known of the auxons of the vitamin B complex. They are found mainly in yeast, and in whole or crushed cereal grain. They may be heated to 160°C. without losing their potency, but contact with oxygen will destroy them in four to eight weeks. The biological activity of auxons is very similar to that of pantothenic acid. Like pantothenic acid, the auxons appear to hold a key position in cellular metabolism and be absolutely essential in regenerative processes.

To establish the biological value of live, uncooked, food, Pottenger and Simonsen carried out nutrition studies over a period of twenty years, using eight generations of cats. Throughout their lives, some of the animals were fed on unheated milk, and raw meat; the others were given boiled milk and cooked meat.

The animals fed on the unheated food remained healthy, as did their offspring. Those fed on cooked food presented symptoms and signs of mesotrophy. Their progeny were born stunted, with malformed skulls and dentition, and other mesotrophic signs. The third generation produced nothing but monsters and stillbirths. From the fourth generation onwards, the lines began to die out. It required four more generations on live food before their mesotrophic changes disappeared.

Further, when infertile soil was manured with the excretions of the "raw food" animals, plant growth developed; but manuring with the excretions of the "cooked food" animals left the soil infertile.

In Japan, the Kuratsunes, a husband and wife team, arrived at similar conclusions in long-term trials with their own diet. A regime consisting entirely of fresh plant foods reduced the basic metabolic rate and increased physical fitness. The same food taken in cooked form produced anaemia, oedema, and other symptoms of severe dystrophy within a few weeks.

McCarrison (Oxford), Abelin (Berne), and other scientists, have come to the conclusion that a live, fresh diet contains unknown vital substances in addition to the known essential factors, and that these also are essential to maintain health.

The purpose of nutrition is to provide the organism with adequate amounts of all substances required to maintain the function and regeneration of cells. But today's average diet is deficient, lacking above all in such essential factors as vitamins, minerals, and other substances.

A lack of essential factors is not, however, the only deficiency in the modern average diet. It contains a great many foreign substances—for example insecticides, preservatives and "improving" agents, and the products of excessive roasting and other cooking methods. Almost all of these have an inhibitory and destructive effect on enzymes and vitamins, resulting in even further depletion of these essential substances.

Experiments have indicated that the consequences of the disorders due to faulty nutrition may be gradually corrected if a diet of maximum biological value is adopted.

In chronic illness proper nutrition is of paramount importance; the usual nutrition should not be maintained. In diabetes, a diet low in carbohydrates must be given; in rheumatism or kidney stones, an uric acid and oxalic acid-free diet; in liver damage, a protein-enriched liver-protective diet.

In cancer, diet should be free from carcinogenic and cancer-promoting agents: it must be adapted to the pathological metabolic situation of the cancer patient.

A cancer diet has to fulfil certain other requirements. It must be rich in vital substances and contain adequate amounts of high-value and easily digested protein. It must be low in animal fats but rich in those vegetable fats having a high content of vitamin F. It must contain as little fermentable carbohydrates—glucose or glucose-forming carbo-hydrates—as possible. Finally, it must consist predominantly of fresh food. I shall now deal with each of these in turn.

Protein substances form, quantitatively, the most important component of all cells. They are high-molecular organic compounds consisting of multi-link chains of nitrogen-containing amino acids. There are twenty-seven different amino acids, all of them necessary for the synthesis of protein. But twelve of these amino acids cannot be formed in the body; they have to be taken in regularly with the daily meals.

Protein-containing food is therefore of maximum biological value only if these twelve amino acids are present in the correct proportion and in adequate amounts. This requirement is fulfilled, for instance, in wholemeal bread, soya beans, nuts, yeast, eggs, milk and milk products, meat, and fish. We can thus have sufficient quantities of full-value protein substances through a variety of foods. The wide-spread belief that our bodies can acquire high-value protein only through meat is inaccurate.

Approximately one gramme of protein substance per kilogramme of body weight should be taken daily. About one sixth of the weight of cottage cheese curds or lean meat is protein substance. The daily requirement of 60 grammes for a person weighing 60 kilogrammes can therefore be satisfied by about 360 grammes of cottage cheese of lean meat.

Protein from sour milk products is the most easily digested and the most wholesome animal protein. If the protein requirement is covered by meat, much larger quantities of incompletely digested protein are left in the large intestine for subsequent bacterial decomposition than with sour milk products. If there is weak digestion, the blood is inevitably flooded with allergising oligopeptides and polypeptides, with putrefaction toxins such as indol, scatol, cadaverine, putrescine and other necrotoxins, and this is generally much worse after meat meals than after milk or cheese meals.

Although meat and milk protein are largely similar, they differ fundamentally as regards their digestibility, utilisation, and compatibility. As I have indicated, milk protein is digested quickly and builds up mainly to body protein; only relatively modest remnants are transformed into biogenous amines and allergens. On the other hand, a much larger proportion of meat is transformed into putrefaction products which have to be neutralised in the liver. Regular and large meat meals will therefore further the autointoxication.

Any tumour-destroying therapy is accompanied by a "re-intoxication" resulting from necrobioses in the tumour. The excretion of these extremely toxic substances is impeded if at the same time there is an "enterogenic auto-intoxication", and a blockage of the detoxicating and excretory functions of the intestinal mucosa. Since both these conditions are regularly present in cancer patients, as little meat as possible should be eaten during tumour therapy.

As I have said, milk protein can be supplied to the body in the form of cottage cheese, sour milk, or cheese. Two litres of milk have about the same protein as 350 grammes of cottage cheese or lean meat—the approximate daily need of a person weighing 60 kilogrammes. But the dietetic value of the various kinds of milk available today varies considerably, and certain kinds are quite unsuitable for cancer patients.

Fresh milk—sweet milk—is to be avoided because it contains at least during the spring months, growth promoting oestrogens which, within the context of an anti-cancer diet, are undesirable. Sour milk, however, is low in such undesirable growth substances owing to bacterial fermentation, and at the same time it is to a considerable extent retransformed to vital protein, that is, to bacterial protein.

But not all kinds of sour milk are equally suitable. Its biological value is higher the more free dextro-lactic acid and gutobligatory bacteria it contains. Curdled milk contains streptococci which generate the dextro-lactic acid that is physiologically essential to the intestinal flora. Buttermilk is particularly valuable because of its high vitamin content, especially its high orotic acid level, and also because of its special liver-protecting efficacy.

Despite its high lactic acid content, ordinary yoghurt is not entirely suitable for a cancer diet. It may dislodge pathological bacteria quickly from the gut, but it cannot supplant the other kinds of sour milk because the yoghurt germs do not stay in the gut and are excreted.

Sour milk products may be regarded as vital protein providers. Their suitability depends on the type of fermentation, the fat and salt content.

Non-fat cheeses are preferable to fat cheeses. Salt-reduced or salt-free cheeses are better than salty cheeses.

Meat, because of its poor digestibility and unfavourable effect on the intestinal milieu should be reduced in a cancer diet. Certain meats are better than others.

All inner organs (liver, spleen, sweetbread, lung etc.) are superior to muscle meat. Game (venison, wild birds) and grazing animals (mutton, lamb), as well as lean saltwater and freshwater fish, are preferable to all other meat sources. Farm animals (veal, beef, poultry) are the next best. Fattened animals (pig, duck, goose, turkey, rabbit) are quite unsuitable. Pork (including wild boar) and all meat products made from it (ham sausage etc.) should be avoided even in the smallest quantities, because of "pork toxins"—the sutoxins—they contain.

Whether meat is dietetically valuable largely depends on its preparation. For some, cooked and roasted meat tastes better than fresh raw meat, but it has not the same biological value. Smoked meat, including sausage, cured fish etc., whatever its origin, is unsuitable. In smoking, these foods are enriched with antiseptic substances which destroy the flora of the mucous membranes and in addition may contain varying amounts of carcinogens.

Soya beans are richest in protein. Weight for weight, they have double the amino acid nutritive value of lean meat. They contain twenty-seven percent starch, eighteen percent high quality oil with a vitamin F content of about fifty percent, and a high proportion of lecithins, which serve as an active metabolic structure substance of the cell membranes, the mitochondria and the cell nucleus.

Nuts, especially hazelnuts, walnuts and almonds also have a high protein value and in addition, contain on average sixty percent high quality fats rich in vitamin F and lecithins, and free from cholesterol. Groundnuts, despite many valuable contents, are unsuitable for a cancer diet.

Yeast is specifically suitable for the nutrition of cancer patients. It contains numerous components capable of developing cancer-inhibiting and detoxicating effects. Dry yeast, living fresh yeast, and fermenting beer yeast are all suitable, but the living yeasts are distinctly superior to dry preparations in their beneficial effect.

Now let us turn to fats—organic compounds formed by combining a glycerine molecule with three molecules of "fatty acids". Fatty acids are organic combinations which consist of the same elements as the sugars, and differ from them merely in their structure. There are two different kinds of fatty acids: saturated and unsaturated.

Saturated fatty acids join with glycerine to form solid fats which are fully saturated with hydrogen atoms and therefore no longer capable of chemical reaction; they are "dead" fats. Unsaturated fatty acids, are not fully saturated with hydrogen, and are therefore capable of chemical reaction. Combined with glycerine, they form liquid fats—oils.

There are many unsaturated fatty acids. Some are of special biological importance because they are used in the body not only as building materials, and fuel, but also as co-ferments and metabolic elements of the cell. These are thus truly vital substances. The essential highly unsaturated fatty acids, such as linolenic and arachidonic acids, are commonly summarised as vitamin F.

The biological value of a fat is greater the more highly unsaturated fatty acids it contains. Vitamin F is a component of certain lecithins. A lecithin-rich cell differs by its lively metabolism and slag-free interior from a lecithin-deficient cell which is packed with slag substances.

In 1962, Neifakh (USSR) reported tumour tissues contain no essential fatty acids, that is, no vitamin F. Any diet rich in solid fats and low in vitamin F may promote the development of cancer, as shown, inter alia, by Kousmine-Meyer and Budwig.

As I have already said, all animal fats—bacon, lard, suet, butter, clarified butter etc. must be regarded as unsuitable, because of their high cholesterol content. All these cholesterol-rich animal products contain predominantly or exclusively dead solid fats and too little "living" or vitamin F-containing fat.

The vitamin F content of vegetable oils depends on their production and preparation. The highest possible vitamin F content is present only in untreated, cold-pressed, oils. Some with such a high vitamin F content, or containing other oxygen-activating components are: cold-pressed and untreated sunflower oil, linseed oil, soya oil, wheat-germ oil, corn oil and thistle oil (whose vitamin F content may reach eighty percent compared to the three percent in butter), plus health margarine prepared from these oils without heating.

Not all vitamin F-containing oils are suitable. Groundnut oil, although rich in vitamin F and tasty, may be contaminated with "aflatoxin"—the toxic yellow mould frequently seen in groundnuts.

The heating of oils and fats reduces or destroys their vitamin F content because at higher temperatures, vitamin F combines readily with oxygen and becomes saturated, thereby losing its vitamin character. Fats of vegetable origin are also deprived of their vitamin F and biologically devalued if they are subjected to prolonged heat during their production. Intense or prolonged heating of fats can also produce carcinogenic toxicants. Finally, heated fats assume allergising properties. Chronic digestive disorders, including precancerous conditions of various kinds, may be caused by regular consumption of heated fats.

Carbohydrates also merit special attention in an anti-cancer diet. They are substances which, in addition to carbon, contain hydrogen and oxygen in the same proportion as water. There are mono-, di-, and polysaccharide carbohydrates.

Monosaccharide carbohydrates are those with six carbon atoms. They include grape sugar (glucose), fruit sugar (fructose), and sorbite (diabetic sugar), a monosaccharide also occurring in fruit—particularly in rowanberries, the small red berry of the mountain ash—and transformed into fructose in the liver. Monosaccharides require no digestion; they simply enter the blood in solution through the intestinal wall.

Disaccharides such as cane sugar or beet sugar, malt sugar or milk sugar, are chemical compounds of two monosaccharide molecules with twelve carbon atoms. They are reduced to monosaccharides by the disaccharide-splitting enzymes of the pancreas and intestinal mucous membrane, and enter the blood in this form.

Polysaccharides such as starch, glycogen and cellulose, are combinations of numerous molecules of monosaccharides. They are reduced to monosaccharides by the process of polysaccharases and are also absorbed in this form through the intestinal wall.

Healthy cells differ from cancer cells in the way they are able to make use of sugar. Healthy cells, with the aid of the oxygen we breathe, burn monosaccharides into carbon dioxide and water. But cancer cells, lacking the required oxydation ferments, cannot utilise oxygen. In the cancer cell, therefore, sugar can be fermented only by the formation of laevo-lactic acid.

Even so, cancer cells cannot ferment all sugars. Apart from glucose, always present in the body in the form of blood sugar, other mono-saccharides are unusable by the cancer cell owing to its lack of the necessary enzyme system. There are therefore two groups of carbo-hydrates: those fermentable by the cancer cell and thus cancer-promot-ing, and those non-fermentable and thus non-cancer-promoting.

The cancer-promoting sugars include, in addition to glucose, those carbohydrates which under the influence of digestive enzymes can be transformed into glucose, especially malt, cane, and beet sugar. This also applies to non-refined brown sugar as well as to sugar syrup, and all tonics, sweets, and jams made from these sugars.

Whether the cell ferments sugar or burns it up to carbon dioxide and water depends not only on the molecular structure of the sugar but also on the cellular enzyme balance and the metabolic activities depend-ing on it. Many enzymes are vitamin-protein combinations, made up of a co-enzyme (the vitamin) and an apo-enzyme (the nucleoproteid). The normal metabolic and oxydation processes are therefore possible only if the cell is adequately equipped with all vital substances. If the supply of vital substances is insufficient, this creates in the cell an enzyme defect. The cell is no longer able to produce the normal metabolic performance and must confine itself to fermenting the energy-supplying carbohydrates.

It hardly needs saying that the fermentation processes are the more intensive the more sugar is available to the cell; with a high glucose content in the blood, the fermentation will be brisk and with a low blood sugar it will be correspondingly reduced. Unfortunately, the custom is still widespread to inject glucose as a "tonic". This can be disadvantageous for the cancer patient.

Whether and to what extent carbohydrates are pathologically fermented depends also on the form in which they are eaten—whether they are digested as fresh fruit or a mixture of fresh fruit, or as a highly concentrated pure substance, such as commercial glucose, beet or cane sugar or sweets and foods made from these. The rise in the blood sugar level after consumption of such sugar concentrates can, under certain conditions, overload the fermentation system of even a healthy cell, placing it in a state of acute vital substance deficiency and causing metabolic disturbance. Clearly carbohydrates are best taken in the living, fresh state.

The habit of eating sweets or of sweetening food and drink with sugar may be dangerous to health. Within a biologically acceptable cancer diet, this habit should be given up, but if that proves too difficult, it is better to use non-fermentable and therefore non-cancer-promoting sugars in preference to commercial sugar.

Fruit sugar is non-fermentable and also develops a specific effect on the liver, but it should be taken only in connection with the necessary vitamins not contained in the pure concentrates of these sugars. In other words, when fruit sugar is taken, it must be complemented with vitamins from another source, for instance from untreated and un-heated honey. Such honey is a vital sugar which, if of good quality, consists of two-thirds fruit sugar and one-third glucose, plus many valuable vital substances.

Milk sugar (beta-lactose), a disaccharide occurring solely in milk and whose fermentative breakdown produces galactose and glucose, is an absolutely vital component of our daily food; many biologically important processes can best function with the aid of milk sugar. It is indispensable for the maintenance of the flora of the small intestine as well as the coli flora of the large intestine. Galactose is required constantly in large quantities for the biosynthesis of many cell components. For these reasons a daily intake of milk sugar should be an essential part of any diet.

Starch—a polysaccharide created by the chemical combination of many monosaccharides—is reduced to monosaccharides in the gut and absorbed in the blood. The starch in bread, puddings, cakes and pastry as well as in starchy vegetables, such as potatoes, is a basic part of almost everyone's daily food. As with meat dishes, the health value of starchy food depends largely on its preparation. Taken as wholemeal, grain is a food of incomparable perfection. One litre of living wheat grain and a pinch of sea salt formed the daily ration of the Roman soldier. Besides containing starch, fats of the highest biological value, living enzymes, and other irreplacable vital substances, 100 grammes of wholemeal wheat even contains protein of full biological value in an amount corresponding to that of about 80 grammes of lean meat. As much as possible of the daily starch intake should therefore be taken in the form of living wholemeal muesli.

Regrettably, nowadays grain is normally eaten neither as wholemeal nor in a living state. It has usually been finely ground, thereby releasing its non-mealy components (bran) and thus the vitamins and minerals. To this "refined" flour are then added insecticides, and bleaching and colouring agents. With this kind of adulturated food, health can be impaired. In this regard, I recommend cancer patients should choose a diabetic style diet.

The relatively new belief that living or fresh food is of importance to overall health has gained ground in recent years. At least half, but better still, two-thirds of each meal should consist of such food.

Abnormal fermentation processes can be prevented by eating fresh food. Among other things, raw fruit and vegetables and their juices, raw wholemeal, raw wholemeal flakes, wheatgerm, non-heated sour milk, cottage cheese, cheese, uncooked sauerkraut and raw egg-yolk are some examples.

Fresh fruit and fresh vegetables are the most easily digested foods we know, passing quickly from the stomach to the gut. But even these can cause flatulence and stomach pains if there is an enzyme deficiency and disturbance of the intestinal flora. In such cases, patients tend, quite wrongly, to blame the food rather than any deficient function in their body. This discomfort can usually be prevented by eating the fresh food either by itself as a separate meal, or as the first course of a meal. If eaten together with or after things hard to digest, for instance meat or potatoes, fresh food will lie on the stomach.

Any fresh food must be chewed deliberately and thoroughly.

The intake of water is also important; the adult human body consists of sixty-five percent water. Even without strenuous exercise, at least one-twentieth of this is lost daily and has to be constantly replaced. The temperature of the air naturally affects the amount of perspiration. But food consumption also has an effect: the more food eaten, the higher the water requirement of the body. How important it is to maintain the water balance can be judged from the fact that a healthy person can survive for four to six weeks without solid food, but usually only six to ten days without water.

The solid slag substances produced in the body can be excreted by the liver, gut, skin, and kidneys, only with the aid of water. The more slag substances produced, the more water is needed for their excretion. Since the slag concentration in urine and perspiration cannot rise above a certain maximum, an insufficient intake of water can cause a congestion of slag and many attendant disorders, even in a person who is fit. A person who is ill and has an increased slag production will be unable to resist the problem if he lacks water nourishment.

As we know, the non-excreted refuse will be deposited in the store cells of the connective tissue. Sooner or later this may cause a mesenchymal blockage leading to failure in the defence mechanisms.

An inadequate intake of fluids can cause many other disorders. The amount of circulating blood, its metabolic functions and the organic functions depending on it are reduced. The blood becomes thicker. The heart has to work harder to keep this thickened blood circulating. The secretion of digestive juices in the salivary glands, liver and gut becomes insufficient. Inadequate indigestion and resorption, and increased intestinal putrefaction with auto-intoxication from the gut are the inevitable consequences.

Research has shown that a healthy person with a normal life-style requires daily 40–50 millilitres of water per kilogramme of body-weight. Therefore a person weighing 60 kilogrammes needs about 3 litres of water every day to preserve the water balance. Since the average daily food intake includes about $1-1\frac{1}{2}$ litres of water, at least another $1\frac{1}{2}-2$ litres of pure water must be supplied. Only half of this necessary amount is taken in by most people. Without knowing it, the average person suffers from dehydration due to a chronic water deficiency.

In order to reduce an already existing excess of slag or to prevent it from developing, it is advisable, unless medically ordered not to for specific reasons, to drink daily in addition to the usual soups and other fluid dishes, between meals—and definitely not with meals—at least two litres of unsweetened herb tea or pure, chlorine-free spring water, perhaps made more tasty with a little fruit juice.

Commercial salt taken from a saltpit is almost pure sodium chloride— it is not balanced with calcium, potassium, and magnesium and other trace elements—and is undesirable from a health point of view.

In preference to saltpit salt, sea salt should be used because it contains all the necessary salt substances in a mixture similar to that found in blood.

But even salts from the sea should not be used to excess. If there is an exaggerated desire for salt, it must be counteracted by using other sorts of seasoning—green herbs and seasonings of high biological value.

Many commercial foods, such as bread, cheese, preserves, meat and sausage products, are treated with saltpit salt during manufacture, and therefore the average diet contains a considerable quantity of such hidden salt which is eaten unwittingly. However, as many foods are also available salt-free or with sea salt, obviously these products are superior and preferable.

Protein, fat and carbohydrates as well as other nutrients in food are transformed by the digestive processes into low-molecular water-soluble compounds which, in watery solution react either acidically or basically. Thus they can alter the chemical reaction of the body fluids in the acidic or basic sense. Since the body can only function normally when the reaction of juices is more or less balanced, a constant supply of only acidic or basic food would be harmful. Clearly, we should endeavour to ensure that the "acid-base equilibrium" is maintained by a correct choice of food.

This equilibrium can only come about if the body is supplied with "base formers" and "acid formers" in balanced proportions with every meal (M. Bircher-Benner, R. Berg, Lahmann et al). Base-formers are all kinds of vegetables and fruit—except those listed below—and all milk dishes. Acid-formers are all cereals and flours, puddings, bread and cakes made from them; sprouts, artichokes, mushrooms, legumes, nuts, cranberries, plums; all fats and oils; eggs and egg dishes, cottage cheese and cheese, and all kinds of meat and fish.

The acid-base equilibrium can be ensured if each meal consists in weight of eighty percent base-formers and twenty percent acid-formers.

All the body's vital processes are subject to a sun-dependent daily rhythm (Forsgren et al); the various vital functions show a rhythmic increase and decrease in activity depending on the time of day. In my opinion, it is wise to tailor our eating habits to these biocosmic rhythms.

Since the protein-digesting power of the gastro-intestinal juices is greatest around noon, protein-containing food should be eaten mainly in the morning and at midday (Hay). The evening meal should be limited mainly to raw salads, fruit, muesli and similar dishes low in protein and calories.

10

Help for the Helpless

IN 1970 SOME OF THE WORLD'S MOST RESPECTED ONCOLOGISTS PUBLISHED a book about cancer that was specifically aimed at a lay audience. That in itself was unusual. Even more remarkable were the admissions their book contained about the effectiveness of the current methods of treating malignant disease.

Sir John Bruce, Professor of Clinical Surgery at Edinburgh University, Scotland, said it should not be assumed that he, or any other surgeon, was satisfied with the contribution surgery had made to managing cancer, that "the future lies elsewhere than in the operating room." Sir John was echoing similar remarks made years before. In 1931, C. Henschen, Medical Director of the Department of Surgery at the University Hospital in Basle, had stated that cancer was a systemic disease, and that therefore it was necessary to use systemic medical treatment as well as surgery. A few years later, Franz Koenig, another eminent surgeon, said: "The curing of cancer is not exclusively a question of surgical techniques; it depends, to a decisive extent, on the condition of the body's defence." In 1938, F. Sauerbruch took a similar line: "We surgeons know we are merely removing the gross anatomical defect, but this does not have any affect on the disease as such."

As for radiology, in 1970, Dr. Eric Easson, Chairman of the Commission of Cancer Control of the International Union Against Cancer in Geneva conceded that from "a purely technical point of view" it was hard to imagine any further significant improvement. Dr. John Q.

Matthias, consultant physician at the Royal Marsden Hospital, London, writing on chemotherapy, admitted cancer could only rarely be cured by drugs.

This frankness is refreshing and to be welcomed. Of more immediate importance, such honesty answers the question as to why those patients whose cancer is either operable or susceptible to irradiation should also be treated by whole-body therapy.

The growth of a tumour—be it a primary tumour, a recurrent growth, or a metastasis—always presupposes two factors:

1. The presence of a tumour milieu and a lowered resistance, with a disposition towards the production of a tumour.
2. The presence of cancer cells which are able to multiply.

These factors cannot be removed either by surgery or radiotherapy.

In theory, radical surgery aims at the complete removal of all cancer cells from the body. Such an aim can rarely, if ever, be achieved because cancer cells continuously emigrate even from the smallest micro-carcinoma. Mathé, Wrba and other researchers have shown in animal studies that even after the most perfect operation—and following radiotherapy—*several million cancer cells still remain in the body*.

Even if it were possible to remove them all, secondaries might still occur because cancer cells are also transmitted by cell-free filtrates, for instance, the contents of squashed tumour cells or blood flowing through the tumour. These fluids contain ultravisible microbes, which may, at any time, trigger the production of new cancer cells in a host whose resistance has been seriously impaired, by such factors as the after-effects of major surgery or an intensive course of radiotherapy.

In 1962, Rubin and other workers, reported that the life expectancy and prospects of a cure for those patients who are either operable or suitable for radiology was directly related to their residual resistance. Those with a strong residual defence system responded well to surgery and were often cured. Those with a weakened resistance, in marked contrast, showed a poor response, and later, clear indications of recurrence. Rubin concluded that, in effect, the fate of a patient as far as a cure went, was decided *before* conventional treatment by the state of the patient's resistance; if that was impaired to the point where it could no longer cope, even the most skilled surgical or radiological intervention would surely fail.

Clearly such a situation is unacceptable to both the patient and doctor. If a cure is not to be a matter of chance, certain steps must be carried out immediately before and after surgery or radiotherapy. These measures are specifically aimed at preventing recurrences by ensuring that the organism's defence system is activated and encouraged to resume its natural role.

Recurrences that do occur after conventional treatment cannot be attributed to any lack of technical expertise on the part of the surgeon or radiotherapist. They have usually worked as well as possible within erroneous terms of reference which state that cancer is a localised disease. But long-term remission can be best achieved, if the *causes* are removed—by whole-body therapy. Careful eradication of the tumour is not enough. Such intervention must always be followed by a treatment regime designed to remove the tumour milieu and to strengthen the body's defence.

No patient who has undergone surgery or radiotherapy, however successfully, should be considered cured. "Cure" is a word which must be used circumspectly in relation to cancer; there is no way of being absolutely sure that all malignant cells are eliminated by any form of (standard) treatment, and, as is well known, in certain malignancies undoubted secondaries or metastases may declare themselves fifteen or twenty years after an apparent cure (Matthias). To avoid that situation, in my view it is essential that every patient, following operation or irradiation, should receive whole-body therapy as outlined in this book.

Yet, as I have said before, surgery has important roles to play. They can be summarised:

1. Surgery is the only method to immediately remove the tumour.
2. Surgery is an essential emergency measure when there is a danger of haemorrhage or other acute threats arising from the tumour.
3. Surgery is an effective means to arrest the toxic effects resulting from the dissolution of the tumour.
4. Surgery will assist detoxication and aid instantly the defence forces of the body.

Because of this, surgery will always be important within the whole-body framework—but with a significant difference. The surgeon will no longer be expected to try to eliminate the sum total of cancer cells. Instead he will concentrate his skills on maintaining and enhancing the host's endogenic defence. Rubin said it very well when he argued in 1962 that the surgeon's objective should be removing as many onco- genic substrates as possible, thus improving the curative powers of the host; that can only be realised when the autogenous defence is still active and when surgery does not further reduce its potency.

Indeed, there is a need for a re-evaluation of all the traditional diag- nostic and therapeutic procedures because, at present, they can con- stitute increased risks for cancer patients. It is now known that even ordinary gynaecological examination in cases of cancer of the uterus or the palpation of nodules in the breast may lead to spreading of cancer cells. The same applies to biopsies carried out for diagnostic purposes. Often these biopsies are dispensable because histological examination can be performed following surgical removal of the tumour. Again, even manual examination of a tumour should be carried out carefully. Squeezing of tissues should be avoided as far as possible, because this may produce a massive dissemination of cancer cells. And surgery should always be limited to the very minimum, so reducing operative stress which can only further weaken the natural defence mechanism.

It must never be forgotten that surgery *at any stage* constitutes certain well-defined risks, such as cardiovascular failure or embolism— along with the ubiquitous threat of dissemination of cancer cells. For these reasons as well, it is absolutely essential that prior to surgery and following it, whole-body measures should be carried out. This is especially vital in cases of lung and other organ resection. When surgery is recommended the following steps should be instituted:

1. Pre-operative whole-body therapy should be a priority so that the internal milieu and resistance are improved. This will diminish the surgical risks.
2. Then the tumour should be removed.
3. Extensive whole-body follow-up therapy should be given until the actual *cause* of the tumour has been cured.

Such steps would dramatically increase the percentage of patients free of clinical disease after treatment. These measures would help to keep in the forefront of the therapist's mind the fact that cancer is not merely a tumour, but a tumour milieu which determines the growth and virulence of it, as well as a lowering of endogenous defence. The therapeutical pattern suggested above is designed to control the virulence of both milieu and tumour, while at the same time the host's resistance is strengthened. It is even possible for an apparently inoperable tumour to become operable after pre-treatment. Thus the overall effect is to offer the optimal chance of a cure.

All this may be achieved by diligent attention to removal of foci, by a reasonably programmed dietary regime and by specific measures aimed at detoxication of the organism. The surgeon will then be able to perform his task secure in the knowledge that his patient has been prepared as far as humanly possible for operation. He can proceed, knowing that three major hazards have been minimised:

1. Peritumoural inflammation, which is often extensive and makes it hard to differentiate between malignant and non-malignant tissue no longer exists.
2. Danger of thrombosis and embolism will be greatly reduced.
3. Surgical shock will be diminished, as will the risk of surgery generally.

The longer surgery can be postponed to allow pre-treatment measures to take effect, the better. But it need hardly be said that in acute situations, surgery must be given precedence over all else. In such cases, operation must be immediately followed by intensive whole-body follow-up measures.

My own observations, coupled with those of many other doctors, show that the use of whole-body therapy before and after surgery increases the expectation of cure to over eighty percent. In other words, eight out of every ten patients who receive this combined treatment may survive five, ten, fifteen years and longer.

Recommendations made for operable cancer are equally valid for those cases recommended for radiotherapy. By removing the tumour from the body in "one go", the surgeon certainly improves local and general symptoms, and takes the pressure off the defence mechanism. Although radiotherapy also destroys the tumour, its break-up by this means leads to massive toxicosis, with all the effects on the milieu and resistance this implies. The body's defence is burdened even more by the damage caused to the connective tissue system by the ionising radiation. This inhibition, leading to a mesenchymal blockage, may last for months. As Wrba wrote: "Every thing that is done to the cancer (by radiotherapy or chemotherapy) is also done to the host."

We have already discussed the efficacy and limits of radiotherapy. It therefore becomes clear that supplementary whole-body therapy is even more vital in such cases.

The radiotherapist should administer the minimum possible dosage while at the same time recognising that whole-body therapy has the important dual role of increasing the sensitivity of the tumour to X-rays and increasing the host's tolerance to them. This can be improved by the administration of a number of specific drugs; clinical experience shows that even tumours initially non-susceptible to radiotherapy may then become responsive. Again, a course of whole-body therapy before irradiation guarantees that the patient will be rid of toxicosis and thus better able to withstand and tolerate the treatment.

Alas, even whole-body therapy cannot totally prevent further deterioration of the milieu or of the already, often extensively, lowered resistance. That is a factor always to be considered, and one more reason for administering the minimum possible X-ray dosage.

As I have said, following a course of such treatment, the general condition of a patient will be poorer than in those who have undergone surgery. Radiotherapy, however small the dose, is bound to create a deterioration in resistance. It is because of this that follow-up whole-body therapy is mandatory—and the earlier the better. Clinical experience indicates that by adopting this approach of using whole-body therapy as a pre- and post-treatment with radiotherapy, the prospects of survival and, even cure, are markedly improved.

What happens in practice is far different. Patients are usually operated and irradiated without the benefit of supportive whole-body therapy. For a time they often feel well within themselves and are persuaded that they have achieved genuine remission. Then their hopes are dashed when fresh tumours occur which are no longer amenable to standard methods. These patients then become "incurable". The tragedy, as my own case files show, is that so many of these cases need not be incurable. They are the ones—and throughout the world there are millions more like them—who have become the victims of what I regard as the Seven Deadly Sins of Cancer:

1. The "charitable" white lie, in which the doctor keeps the diagnosis of cancer from his patient, is without doubt the most deadly of all these "sins". Withholding the truth, apart from being ethically dubious, also means that a patient cannot become involved in the

essential two-way partnership with his physicians that allows curative measures to achieve the maximum effect.

2. Equally wrong is the "sin" encompassed in the oft-heard arguments of many doctors that whole-body therapy, either as a pre- or post-treatment to other methods, is not necessary. To reinforce their case they argue further that, in the case of surgery, the operation has been radical, that the "accepted" way of "curing" cancer has been achieved, and that there is no need for any other treatment. Similar arguments are applied to radiotherapy. The patient and his relatives are left in a state of induced euphoria which is too-often shattered when the disease returns.

3. The third deadly "sin" is ignorance of the role that whole-body therapy as a follow-up treatment can play. Coupled with this is the further misapprehension about the very meaning of follow-up treatment. The popular idea of follow-up treatment after surgery is to order a course of radiotherapy. But, at best, this is no more than a tumour-specific measure which does not have any part in treating the actual cause of the cancer. Yet, to succeed, any follow-up treatment must attack the source and the actual cause of the cancer to avoid metastases and secondaries recurring. That is the avowed aim of whole-body therapy—and happily there are many cases who can testify to its success. This therapy is the only means available of returning the abnormal metabolic milieu to normal so that the host can recognise and destroy cancer cells already existing or in the process of formation. Further, this method allows for an actual cure of the disease by removing the host's predisposition to produce tumours.

4. The fourth deadly "sin" is the widely-held belief that proper follow-up treatment does exist within the framework of conventional medicine. In practice this turns out to be routine "check-ups", in themselves necessary because over fifty percent of all those who have survived surgery and radiotherapy have, in fact, a high chance of contracting secondaries. The "follow-ups" are designed in the hope that such recurrences can be discovered at an early stage. It is true that metastases may be discovered during such a check-up. But it is equally true that the check-up has not *prevented* the secondaries appearing. And, by the time they are found, the patient is often deemed as beyond further treatment. The tragedy of these check-ups is that they lull the patient, and sometimes his physician, into a false

state of well-being. Worst of all, the patient too often believes the check-up is actually some kind of preventive treatment. It is nothing of the kind.

5. The fifth deadly "sin" is the belief that a few weeks' holiday is beneficial following surgical or radiological treatment. It is certainly pleasant to have such a rest after a spell in hospital. But the time should be applied to the far more urgent and important matter of undergoing positive whole-body aftercare. Those days and weeks following an operation or irradiation are, as we have seen, crucial for a patient's long-term survival. This is *not* the time to lie on a beach or potter about in the sun. This *is* the time to strengthen a patient's bodily defence. Too often, a period of blissful convalescence is followed by the discovery that the cancer has returned, and that the patient is about to be consigned to the category of incurables.

6. The sixth deadly "sin" is performed by those doctors who urge patients who have undergone conventional treatment to go on special diets designed to fatten them. Now, it is common knowledge that over-eating is harmful even for healthy people. The idea that people ought to weigh as many kilogrammes as they measure in centimetres exceeding one metre is a fallacy long disproven. Actuarial statistics repeatedly show that life expectancy is reduced by a year for each kilogramme of overweight. A person who is say, twenty pounds overweight, can expect to live ten years less than one who is not. It is doubly wrong then to pump food into cancer patients in the belief that it will "build them up to go out into the world strong and healthy". Numerous experiments have shown that such feeding, far from increasing bodily resistance, lowers it—and so contributes to recurrences. Further proof of this can be seen in the cancer statistics for the two World Wars. During the war years the numbers dropped significantly; one reason for this was the fact that cancer patients, like everybody else, were kept on reduced rations. My own clinical observations show that a pronounced weight increase is a triggering factor in the development of metastases.

7. The seventh deadly "sin" is to recommend whole-body therapy as a follow-up—and then fail to see that this is carried out properly and that a patient has all the benefits accruing from such treatment. The problem is one of education; a realisation that it is not enough to pick and choose from a carefully-tailored programme. The whole regime must be followed through. For instance, it is virtually

useless to lay down dietary rules—and then neglect to deal with foci. All the measures within whole-body therapy are framed to interlock and complement each other. Partial treatment is not enough.

By removing these "sins" a major step would have been undertaken in coping with that most important of all problems—that of the so-called "incurable" cancer patient.

"Incurable" is a word that is rarely heard among medical men. It makes most doctors quite uncomfortable to even think about it, let alone speak it. For it is a word which makes it tragically clear how limiting surgery, radiotherapy and chemotherapy are in the management of cancer. The vast number of patients I have treated have all progressed beyond such treatments. It must never be overlooked that only about twenty percent of all conventionally treated patients suffering from cancer, including cancer of the skin, live for five years or more after surgery, irradiation and chemotherapy. Despite improvements in technique, a decisive increase in this percentage cannot be expected in the present state of knowledge. For the remaining eighty percent of all cancer patients who receive treatment, present methods cannot offer even a five-year remission.

There are a number of reasons why neoplastic conditions cannot always be successfully treated by surgery or irradiation, and so are designated incurable.

At the onset of neoplastic development there are, tragically, no symptoms in most cases. And even in advanced malignancy the symptoms are not often obvious. Because of this perniciously insidious development the majority of patients undergo treatment when little can be achieved. Cancer is regarded as incurable when the affected organ cannot be completely removed because of its vital significance to the host, or if a tumour has spread so far that radical removal is no longer possible. This is often the case with tumours of the brain, the liver, the bile ducts and the pancreas, or tumours which have invaded major blood vessels. Very often, distant metastases in the skeleton, the lungs or other organs are already present by the time a diagnosis is made. This leads to what is then described as "primary incurability"—a situation where nothing can be done, in conventional terms, following diagnosis.

Primary incurability also exists if other diseases are present with cancer, such as cardiovascular conditions; in such cases surgery or irradiation are regarded as too risky. Statistically, about two thirds of all cancer patients must be considered primarily incurable at the time of diagnosis. For the remaining one third surgery and radiotherapy offer some prospects of a cure. But these methods are symptomatic. Experience shows the majority of patients treated conventionally develop secondaries. Often these cannot be further treated. This leads to what is known as "secondary incurability".

If these cases are included, the total number of incurable cancer cases is nearly eighty percent. In other words, eight out of every ten cases of diagnosed cancer can expect no lasting help from surgery, radiotherapy or chemotherapy, as these methods are applied today.

But two things need to be clearly understood:

1. Surgeons generally regard cases as *incurable* when a tumour has invaded vital organs or when metastases have occurred, and neither can be removed. But these cases should be classed only as *inoperable*.
2. Many inoperable tumours may still respond satisfactorily to radiotherapy. But if they do not, radiologists tend to describe them as incurable. However, they are merely not curable by radiotherapy.

From this it will be seen that the accepted definition of incurability is no longer valid. It has been out-moded by the fact that there is a third way available—whole-body therapy. There can be no justification for abandoning those millions of patients who have been given up as incurable.

With the so-called incurables—as indeed with those cases which do initially respond to conventional treatments—whole-body therapy includes two basic aims:

1. Removing as much of the tumour as possible, even rendering inoperable tumours operable, or susceptible to radiotherapy.
2. Removal of malignant disease from the organism as a whole by means of a specific, causal, therapy.

These two aims are not mutually exclusive. They must always be used together, to complement each other. Again, tumours which cannot be treated by a classic routine may still respond to immunotherapy, chemotherapy or enzyme therapy. And all these measures have the maximum effect if they are co-ordinated within the framework of the whole-body therapy.

For obvious reasons this method is slower to show results than surgery. Restoring the bodily defence can take months, often many months. Results may only be achieved if natural resistance is to some extent present, and if it can be re-activated and strengthened by medical treatment. But, in my experience, even in the most advanced cases, this quite often happens—patients who appeared beyond help have responded surprisingly well. It is interesting to note that those with other chronic illnesses such as rheumatism, diabetes, and even cirrhosis of the liver, in addition to cancer, have been relieved and sometimes cured by whole-body therapy, proving yet again that this combined treatment is a truly causal one.

This book has been written for the so-called incurables: the majority of cancer patients given up by the localists as hopeless cases. They are incurable in the conventional way. They need not be incurable if the wholebody regime including immunotherapy is applied. In 1953, I wrote that the "cancer problem can only be solved if we find a cure for the incurable". Today, I believe whole-body therapy opens the way to just that solution. There is still a long way to go, but already it offers real help for the helpless.

Twenty-five years of clinical experience with over 8,000 cases of all types of cancer offered me an opportunity to evaluate the effectiveness of whole-body and immunotherapy. I have regularly published my observations, treatment methods and statistical studies. These studies indicate that genuine remissions have been achieved in a wide variety of cancers. The publications are listed in the bibliography.

All the patients selected for statistical analysis could be properly termed in the medical sense as being beyond conventional treatment. During the preparation of the surveys it was mandatory to check the histology of every patient. All previous treatment was correlated.

Results of whole-body and immunotherapy were also independently analysed by Audier and Korthoff of Leiden University, Holland. They reviewed 252 cases from a random sample of 750 patients. Of these 252 patients, 42 (16·6) percent were alive and fully fit for work five years later.

Among subsequent studies I analysed 370 patients, who were given the combined whole-body and immonotherapy as a follow-up treatment shortly after surgery or radiotherapy. Of these patients 322 (87 percent) are alive and well after a period of five years, with no relapses or detectable cancer. Thus with this kind of follow-up treatment the danger of relapse, which according to the World Health Organisation statistics is 50 percent, can be reduced to 13 percent.

11

Prevention is better than Cure

ONE OF THE MOST STARTLING STATISTICS RESULTING FROM THE PAST fifty years of cancer research is that eighty percent of all cancer is caused by the interaction between the individual and the environment in which he lives. Writing specifically about Great Britain, but equally applicable to other industrialised countries, Richard Doll has stated that with proper control of our environment, "we might now be able to prevent about forty percent of the cancer deaths that occur annually in men, and a somewhat smaller proportion—about ten percent in women."

Well, what are these harmful environmental factors which might be controllable, or avoided?

Some of the better known occupationally-induced carcinomas are the lung cancer of vintners (caused by inhalation of sprays containing arsenic); of workers in uranium mines, in asbestos and chrome works; cancer of the bladder of aniline workers; and the multitude of cancers caused by tar, soot, pitch, mineral oil etc.

The frequency of occupationally-induced cancer has already been considerably reduced by stricter factory regulations. Expenditure in this field has begun to pay a handsome dividend.

At least fifteen times more smokers than non-smokers are killed by cancer of the bronchi. Since World War II, the incidence of smoking among women has greatly increased and helped to swell the gruesome statistics. According to Gabka (1970), the true rate of cure for treatment of lung cancer by surgery and radiation is only one percent. Prevention is clearly of extreme importance.

It is quite simple: cigarette smoking should be given up. Simply to reduce the consumption is not sufficient; it has to be stopped altogether. If not, the end product will continue to be more deaths.

Removal of cancerogenic compounds entering the atmosphere from the chimneys of certain kinds of factories is recognised as one of the most urgent health tasks. In industrial areas, smoke sometimes filters out ninety percent of the ultraviolet rays from the sun.

On motorways, exhaust gases poison adjoining fields; two grammes of lead can be present in 100 grammes of the grass verge.

The continuing nuclear tests in the atmosphere pollute the air, water, fields and meadows, and the animals.

The abuse of drugs contributes to our being swamped by poisons, leading to an increased incidence of cancer. More symptoms are caused by drugs than they are by disease; Kümmerle's text-book on the side-effects of drugs is a fatter tome than most text-books on internal medicine.

The damaging effect of high tension wires, of subterranean streams and of other geopathic stimuli which alter the bio-electric field to which normal vital functions are coupled, have been discussed for decades, and have been confirmed experimentally.

In addition to the physical stresses, we all face mental stress during our lives.

Fudalla, in his book "The Present as Patient", lists many of the mental stresses caused by our civilisation. Friction in our public working life, or in our private family life, can impose a severe burden on the organism; if it continues too long, it may damage or even completely destroy the defence forces of the body. Bahnson has published summaries on the connection between psyche and cancer; only by a conscious effort to reduce stress may the pathological effects stemming from it be prevented.

Every effort should be made to react to personal problems in as relaxed a manner as possible. The more pleasure a person is able to feel, and to give, the more he is able to look with detachment at the unalterable every day problems, the easier will solutions result for apparently insoluble tensions. Negative attitudes have negative effects on the body. A person who is reasonably free from anxiety and aggression will be better able to overcome mentally and physically the dangers and difficulties of life.

Many people believe health can be achieved by eating expensively; they eat only the best food, attractively prepared, and as much as possible. This they wash down with expensive alcoholic drinks into a body which is already overtaxed. A more sensible diet would prevent a good deal of injury. Of course, such advice, as I know from personal experience, is easier to give than to accept. Nevertheless, even Hippocrates knew that "your food is your medicament, your medicament your food."

Everyone should try to establish a proper balance between work, leisure, and sleep. A large part of our free time should be spent in the outdoors; we should sleep and work with the windows open, and from time to time, consciously breathe deeply.

Too little attention is paid to the skin as a "third kidney". Its ability to excrete poisons should be stimulated by promoting the blood flow and by active as well as passive production of perspiration. Active production of sweat by sports and exercise is much better than passive production by sauna and other hyperthermic means. Proper renal excretion is furthered by taking plenty of fluid between—and not with —meals.

Health spas should not be thought of simply as fashionable expressions of a prosperous society. If possible, they should be visited twice a year, and supported by a fast or a fruit diet day once a week.

In my opinion, we should give more attention to the harmful exchange of electrical charges between the organism and clothing. Natural raw materials—leather, wool, natural silk, cotton, linen—are much superior to artificial materials. They are semi-conductors, whereas artificial materials are all non-conductors. Semi-conductors will permit the natural exchange of charges between body and environment; they prevent the static charges arising between clothes and skin. They also ensure proper breathing of the skin and prevent accumulation of heat. Natural materials should also be preferred for carpets, soft furnishings, and bed linen. Palm (1968), Kaufmann (1967), and others have described in detail the damage caused by modern building methods using artificial, "non-breathing" materials which change and deflect the bio-electric field.

It has been said that a person may either live so that he apparently unavoidably stumbles into disease, or be aware of his ability to maintain or improve health and resistance (Kötschau). If, however, resistance has already been weakened by internal or external causes, precancerosis should be recognised by true early diagnostic measures so that neoplasms may be prevented by specific internal treatment. Additionally, a doctor should be consulted immediately if any of the following suspicious symptoms are noticed:

> Any change in a wart or mole; an ulcer that will not heal; a nodule in the breast or in any other part of the body; unusual haemorrhages or discharges from bodily openings; persistent discomfort of the upper abdomen, or any persistent change of the normal intestinal function; difficulties in swallowing; persistent hoarseness and cough; any neurological symptoms that are increasing and for which no cause can be found. In fact any suspicious changes in the body should be investigated immediately.

Self-examination by women is particularly important. Those who do not carry out regular self-examinations should be instructed on the method by their doctors. As well as any lump in the breast, a drawing-in of the skin or the excretion of fluid or blood from the nipple may be important early symptoms of cancer. These latter are not accompanied by any further indications in the early, curable, stages. I have found over and over again among female patients that in spite of extensive publicity they had neglected these early symptoms and had thus reduced their chances of cure. Obviously, if there is irregular bleeding or discharges, gynaecological examination is a must.

Measures designed to prevent disease are much less complicated and more promising than curative measures. On the basis of this a new discipline of medicine has been developed with the aim of finding new means of preventing disease, especially the chronic diseases. Early recognition of cancer, and solving the problem of cardiovascular disease and rheumatism are three of the major aims in this field.

K. H. Bauer, in his book "The Cancer Problem", has underlined the importance of the "triple early": early recognition, early diagnosis, and early treatment. During the last few decades, this has been the *leitmotif*, the guiding principle, in the fight against cancer. But despite the great efforts made, the results so far have been largely disappointing. Nevertheless, the efforts ought to be continued.

One reason for the lack of success may be found in the general attitude of the population. Many people do not dare go to the doctor for fear the disease they already suspect or recognise may be con-firmed.

In the United States, about forty-four thousand women develop uterine cancer each year; annually, some fourteen thousand die of the disease. Health administrators in America, Britain and elsewhere repeatedly draw attention to the necessity for regular and early diagnos-tic examinations. Their warnings are often ignored.

Today the chances of cure in the early stages of cancer of the cervix are much improved, and it can be diagnosed by the PAP cervical smear test developed by the American oncologist George Papanicolaou. He discovered it was not necessary to surgically remove tissue to show a possible threat from cancer, and his PAP test is now widely used. It is simple, quite painless, and quick. As it is also harmless, it may be used without fear not only in apparently healthy persons, but also on patients where cancer is suspected.

The results of the PAP test can be classified as follows:

PAP I: normal and clearly benign
PAP II: not quite normal, but still benign
PAP III: doubtful, possibly suspect
PAP IV: seriously suspect of cancer
PAP V: malignant

Generally, at stages III to V, conventional medicine carries out conisation, to remove the suspected tissue. But that is not enough: the conisation should be followed by internal preventive treatment in order to remove the primary precancerosis. Even preferable to this, such internal treatment should begin at stage II, possibly preventing transi-tion of the disease into malignancy. Clearly, no one should wait until stage V, when a tumour is manifest, before beginning treatment—although unhappily, this is too often the case. Partly because of this, despite its potential value, the PAP test has only improved the early diagnosis of cancer by two or three percent.

There are many tests which aim to diagnose the presence of a tumour, even if only of microscopic size. As examples, the maligno-lipin test of the Japanese worker Kosaki, and the clostridium test of the Austrian Möse, are useful, but reported to be rather complicated and only become positive when a microtumour exists, wherever it is sited; Abderhalden's Test and the Cytolysis test of Freund and Kaminer, developed by Christiani, also only become positive when a tumour is present.

The value of such tests is undoubted. The whole-body concept of cancer demands, however, that diagnosis should be established at an even earlier date; before the signs of the secondary precancerosis have arisen, before any "trigger" induces formation of tumours. The diagnosis should not be established after the bell has tolled the final act of the disease, but at the latest, "five minutes before midnight", so that transition towards malignancy and tumour formation may be prevented (K. H. Bauer).

Biological, or humoral tests, have this aim. Indeed, for decades researchers have searched for a satisfactory humoral test for primary precancerosis—testing the blood, urine, lymphs etc. There are more than thirty such tests. Many of them, valuable as they are, have not been developed further as they have been judged by localistic concepts—by the wrong parameters.

According to the localist school, a cancer test will become positive only if a tumour is present. Thus, to judge the value of a test, localists ask how early in tumour development does the test demonstrate the presence of cancer. But the cancer disease exists before a tumour forms. Further, localists expect a test should become negative immediately the tumour is removed.

From the whole-body standpoint, quite different criteria apply. An ideal humoral test would be positive at each stage of the cancer disease. Thus in early precancerosis, it would be weakly positive. As the precancerosis progresses, it would become more strongly positive, and be strongest at the stage of tumour development. The test would remain positive after the tumour has been removed, but become slowly negative as the organism regains its resistance to tumour formation following internal treatment. However, if the milieu deteriorates again later, then the test would become positive again, indicating renewed danger, and fresh internal treatment would be started to counter the danger of a recurrence.

If such a humoral test showed a positive result in twenty to thirty percent of apparently healthy people, it should not be regarded as a failure. Rather, it would confirm the practical experience that, statistically speaking, this percentage of healthy people will develop cancer. Localistic diagnosticians might object to such "inaccuracies" in a cancer test. But I share Cardozo's opinion that what matters in cytological diagnosis is not primarily the degree of certainty, but the sensitivity of the method. It would be better to give the likelihood of protection to the twenty to thirty percent of people with a cancer disposition, however scanty the actual evidence may be, than to let even one person die, only because doctors waited until a tumour developed.

It is true that there could not be certain proof that cancer would have resulted had the patient not undergone internal treatment; in theory, if no tumour formed, it might be argued that the test gave the wrong result initially. But evidence for the value of such a test might be provided at the secondary precancerosis stage. If, at this stage, as a patient was suffering relapse after relapse, as a benign neoplasm was moving gradually and inexorably nearer to malignancy—*but* at the last moment was treated by internal therapy, relapses and the transition to malignancy prevented, then there would be strong evidence the test had proven itself.

Naturally, the test could also be used for patients whose cancer had already been treated by surgery or radiotherapy. If the cancer test became negative following internal treatment after the localised treatment, no new tumour should arise. If the test remained positive, because there had been no internal treatment, or not enough, it could be assumed the patient would have recurrences or metastases.

If such a test procedure, and subsequently the treatment of those people who showed a cancer disposition, were generally carried out on the broadest basis, evidence for its correctness would be provided within a few years by a reduction in the number of cancer patients. So long as there is no such recognised cancer test available, I would urge as a basis for cancer prevention the simultaneous use of several existing tests, so that a reliable statement about cancer disposition could be made by means of a summation diagnosis.

In my clinic, I have always carried out several tests contemporaneously, in order to assess their validity. I found two major limitations which affect the informative value of these tests and which have to be taken into account in practice.

The first limitation, though not fatal for the patient, is that of uncertainty. It occurs when the test is positive although there is in fact no cancer; for example, in cases of focal toxicosis. Nevertheless, this result does indicate a sensitisation of the organism with damage to the regulatory and functional mechanism due to the focal toxins. Therefore, although the presence of cancer has not been demonstrated specifically, the test indicates a danger from foci and the need for their removal. If the test remains positive once the foci have been removed, then it indicates the presence of true precancerosis.

The second limitation, a negative result when there is in reality cancer, can be disastrous. It may be due to mesenchymal blocking which is so pronounced that the body is altogether unable to cope with the pathological progress, and thus is unable to record the advance of the disease. Patients with advanced tumours may show a normal blood condition and may present a picture of health. This state of affairs is most deceptive: cancer tests on such patients may remain negative even if metastases are present. They respond poorly to treatment, and may require it for a very long time, so as to remove the mesenchymal blocking. Once the block has been broken through, often following a bout of high fever, the response to internal treatment may be evidenced by an increase of blood sedimentation rate and sudden changes in the blood situation. From then on, cancer tests become positive.

To recapitulate: in my view, preference should be given to discovering a humoral method of early diagnosis of primary precancerosis to ensure true prophylaxis of tumour formation. The efforts now being made to find a means of earlier diagnosis of tumours should be supplemented by attempts to develop a really early diagnosis of the cancer *illness* to prevent tumour formation.

Although this may sound utopian, it is my opinion that further research on these lines could produce worthwhile advances within the foreseeable future. As Morgenstern said, "He who does not recognise the goal will not find the way."

12

Cancer: A Second Opinion

THE ROAD TOWARDS THE CONTROL OF CANCER WE HAVE TRAVELLED in the past chapters has had one recurring signpost, firmly rooted, pointed squarely down that road, towards one essential pre-condition for any success: to destroy the marauding cancer cells a concerted effort must be made to restore the sick body to a level of health by stimulating its own immune responses so that malignancy is overcome by the inherent natural defences.

It can, and often is a hard fight, relentless and demanding, for patient and doctor. But they must fight together. To fail means all else is lost. Most doctors would admit, if only among themselves, that it is the natural healing power of the body which conquers disease. It was Hippocrates who first said: the doctor treats, Nature heals. That much has not changed in two thousand years. But, in the past hundred years, in their very attitude towards cancer, many doctors have forgotten, or neglected, another caveat of Hippocrates: prescribe the best possible treatment for the afflicted. Above all do no harm.

Nobody can deny that harm has been done. Nobody can deny that the classic methods have reached their maximum efficiency. Nobody can deny that more people are contracting cancer.

Yet, it is all so preventable. It need not have happened. It must not continue to happen.

There are some who say that any warning, however reasoned,

however well-meant, however dire, will go unheeded; that any hope of a change in direction in treating cancer is now too late.

I do not agree.

I believe there will be a change, there must be a change, that there already *is* a change. There are many mysteries to be solved, many answers to be found for questions which have puzzled scientists for centuries. But there is little doubt that once again—after a century of advancing deeper into a treatment cul-de-sac—cancer therapy is moving in the right direction. The spur has been immunology; the incentive has been the urgent need to find answers in terms of cancer control to the problems of tomorrow.

Stress, as we now know, can play a role in the development of cancer. It can be a trigger factor. It is on the increase. By 1980, just seven years away when these words were written, it has been estimated that in the United States one in every three adults will be suffering from medically-verifiable stress. Over half of them will be suitable cases for hospitalisation. A similar prognosis can be made for Britain, Germany and other highly-organised, highly-compressed, over-industrialised nations.

Stress is not generally regarded as being of any real importance in cancer. This is not surprising as long as the tumour is held to be all-important.

Nor is another increasing problem of our world usually given sufficient weight in connection with cancer. It is pollution.

Much has recently been written about the need for a co-ordinated ecology plan to cope with the world's pollution problem. Our food gets more processed, more adulterated, more poisoned as we become the victims of clever advertising aimed to convince us that poor-quality, artificially-sweetened, pre-packed, deep-frozen, dehydrated food is *good* for us! The same applies to our drinking water, our beer, our table wines. The air we breathe daily gets dirtier. The environment of some industrial communities is already alarming and could become dangerous. Environmental factors play their part in how and when cancer develops. The warning is clear. Thankfully, it is being heeded: clean-air and pure-food programmes are on the increase. But there is a need for more.

There is also a need for further education which plainly states that much of what is postulated today about cancer treatment is wrong, and that a great deal of what is valuable, constructive and beneficial has been put aside. This has a depressing chain-effect of fear which leads to delay, and, in too many cases, to needless death. Any health education programme must set out the limitations of the classic methods. There must be no sacrificing of truth, the facts must be clearly stated. We must move away from the idea that when the disease has passed beyond the reach of the present methods of classic treatment, all that is left is to see that patients enjoy the final period of their lives as pain-free as possible. Control of pain is, of course, important; nobody should be left with a burden of suspended dying where only a truncated semblance of life is maintained.

But doctors and patients must be alerted that more can be done than merely controlling pain; that a proven treatment exists which views a patient as a *whole*, that seeks, and treats, the *cause* of their illness, that achieves this by combining all that is best in humoral pathology with cellular pathology.

Both are important. Cellular pathology shows changes in the cells and organs, but not always how those changes occur. Humoral pathology not only reveals how and why cellular changes have occurred, but offers co-ordinated ground rules for treatment. By following those rules, it is possible to improve the body's natural defence, allowing, for example, a chance for immunotherapy to work.

The rules of humoral pathology must once again find a place in the teaching curricula. From the day they enter medical school students must also be taught that cancer is a general disease, and is *not* always incurable beyond a certain stage. Surgery and radiotherapy have their place, and a valuable one it is. But they are no more than symptomatic tools.

Nor should our future doctors be encouraged to believe that the all-important objective is to find the *cause* of cancer. It *is* important, but no more than discovering the *cause* of why cancer is still treated the way it is. In some ways treatment itself appears to be *incurable* as long as it sticks to the localistic dogma. In the meantime, people die by the thousands from cancer who need not have died.

But there is a change in the air.

The localistic concept of cancer is being put in perspective, is coming to be recognised as no more than a good, but also a limited, symptomatic approach. The great research centres are mobilising their talent, their money, their influence to examine the definite possibilities that a combination of whole-body therapy and classic therapy holds.

This can never be achieved unless there is a full and frank recognition that the fundamental cancer problem is due to a contradiction of conceptions.

Throughout this book I have tried to make it clear that it is an unwritten law of medicine that the concept of pathogenesis must be the basis of any successful treatment. If later research indicates there are deficiencies in an original concept, then it must be changed; if it is totally wrong, then it must be replaced. This has always been so in medicine. But, in the past century, this rule has not been applied to cancer. The localistic concept has been defended, often fiercely, even though it has been shown to be wrong and misleading. Any real progress can only be achieved if such thinking is finally discarded.

The research centres are showing the way; one scientific paper follows another with the argument that the body's natural resistance plays a decisive part in oncogenesis, regardless of which hypothesis, virus or Mycoplasma etc., is the right one. This seems to confirm that the important factor is to manage the endogenous environment, the milieu. For the cancer-afflicted organism, only one thing matters— recognising the cancer cell and destroying it. Therefore, a successful treatment must be a causal one. Whole-body therapy offers this for every type of malignancy because it is a specific treatment against the tumour and a basic treatment designed to restore the body's natural resistance, whose impairment can be regarded as the cause of every tumour. This combination offers real and long-term results.

Twenty years ago I suggested that a long-term strategy for managing the disease be set up. Mathé, among others, has now confirmed the validity of this suggestion. Research is showing that cancer is a chronic general disease. Therefore, treatment should be primarily in the hands of the whole-body oncologist. It is he who should plan the strategy for patients; and, while continuing with immunotherapy, refer the patient at the appropriate moment to the surgeon or radiotherapist. The whole-body oncologist must always take into account that when the tumour has manifested itself, the host has lost a decisive battle—the struggle of natural resistance against cancer. A wise strategist will not begin treatment with any measures that may destroy any remaining resistance, unless there is no alternative.

Surgery and radiotherapy have their place in this combination; outside it, they are not the ultimate answer to the chronic, systemic disorder that cancer is. Immunotherapy, too, is most effective when used as part of the combination treatment; when applying it, care must also be taken to try and restore the host's own defence, even if more effective immunological agents are developed.

That may take some time. Of immediate concern is the present situation of treatment. In general practice nothing has changed very much for the past decades, apart from the additional application of chemical drugs. Treatment still follows the same pattern; little is done to restore natural resistance, either primarily or as follow-up treatment.

The latest trends in research have yet to be put into practice. This still holds true, in spite of the fact that immunology has been available for some seventy years. It is only now, in its "second coming", that this branch of medicine is being taken note of. But, in view of the virulence of cancer, it is high time that we made immediate, widespread and practical use of immunotherapy *now*—and not wait until we know its infinite working mechanism. Immunotherapy is not toxic. But, on the other hand drugs which are highly toxic are freely prescribed—because their working mechanism is known.

Something, indeed, seems to be very wrong; the control of cancer seems to have moved a long way from that good, old-fashioned yardstick that a treatment was acknowledged as successful if it healed.

No matter how the statistics are presented, nobody can say that the classic methods have solved the cancer problem. The number of "incurables" shows that. I prefer to regard them as "untreatable by classic methods". The fact is that they are still treatable by whole-body therapy combining immunotherapy.

Nevertheless, in terms of treatment, cancer is in that cul-de-sac I mentioned earlier. It needs boldness, courage and an honest recognition that a grave mistake has been made before escape is possible. The medical profession must show the way.

The present-day work in immunology is indicating the direction cancer therapy should take. Immunologists have opened the gate to the whole-body approach in cancer—and indeed all chronic illnesses.

But *every* doctor who has a cancer patient must rethink his attitude towards the disease. He must recognise that there is a need for a properly co-ordinated co-operation between the classic methods and the concept that cancer, from the very outset, is a disease of the whole body.

This is the way to progress if we hope that the cancer statistics of tomorrow will be better than they are today; and that future generations will no longer have to live with the scourge that today needlessly claims so many hapless victims.

Appendix

Appendix

Case history No. 64/50:
Mrs. K. G. (born February 20th, 1909)

TOTAL REMISSION OF RECURRING INOPERABLE UTERINE CANCER

November 1949: Primary inoperable utero-cervical cancer, stage II, histologically verified platy-cullular carcinoma. Remission after radiation.

July 1950: Egg-sized local recurrence. Radiotherapy unsuccessful. Pelvic space walled up with solid cancerous masses; rectal passage totally blocked; palliative colostomy essential. In moribund condition patient admitted to Issels-Klinik.

Condition on admission, October, 1950:
Pelvic and hypogastric spaces totally blocked with large cancer masses adhering to surrounding organs. Bleeding tumour masses emerging from vagina. Patient almost pulseless.

Treatment: Whole-body therapy and immunotherapy.

Result: Disappearance of all tumour symptoms within five months. Twenty-three years have passed without any further signs of detectable cancer.

Case history No. 166/52:

Mrs. Th. C-D. (born September 17th, 1933)

TOTAL REMISSION OF RECURRING PLEURAL SARCOMA

September 1952: Exploratory surgery revealed primary tumour adhering on left chest-wall with ramifications encircling spinal column. Diaphragm covered with metastases. Chest-wall shows carcinomatous infiltration. Sub-total surgery performed. Histopathology: Fibroplastic sarcoma. Palliative follow-up radiotherapy unsuccessful and halted. Prognosis: absolutely hopeless. Patient referred to Issels-Klinik on October 29th, 1952.

Condition on admission:
Medically verified as terminal.

Treatment: Whole-body therapy and immunotherapy.

Result: Complete remission in one year.

In August 1954 massive recurrence in left pleura. No surgery possible. Palliative radiation. No remission.

Re-admission to Issels-Klinik.

Condition on admission:
Massive tumour on left lung, cutaneous metastases on the left chest-wall.

Treatment: Whole-body therapy and immunotherapy.

Result: Complete recovery within two years. Subsequently married, produced two children. After twenty-one years no detectable signs of cancer.

Case history No. 46/53:
Mrs. E. Dr. (born March 6th, 1919)

TOTAL REMISSION OF RECURRING UTERINE CANCER

February 1952: Sub-total extirpation of utero-cervical cancer, stage III. Histopathology: Platy-cellular carcinoma. Follow-up radiation.

August 1952: First relapse. Remission after maximum dose radio-therapy.

February 1953: Second relapse. No further radiotherapy possible. Patient admitted to Issels-Klinik in terminal stage.

Condition on admission, March 1953:
Pelvic space totally walled up with solid tumour masses, vital indication of colostomy because of stenosis of rectum.

Treatment: Whole-body therapy and immunotherapy.

Result: In two years total disappearance of all tumour symptoms. Twenty subsequent years free of detectable cancer.

Case history No. 51/53:

Mrs. S. G. (born June 2nd, 1900)

TOTAL REMISSION OF LUNG METASTASES ARISING FROM PRIMARY BREAST CANCER

Iuly 1952: Right-sided mastectomy because of mammary tumour. Histopathology: Penetrating adeno-carcinoma. Follow-up radio-therapy.

January 1953: Pulmonary metastases both sides. Prognosis hopeless. Patient admitted to Issels-Klinik.

Condition on admission, April 1953:
Multiple pulmonary metastases of varying size. Bad general condition.

Treatment: Whole-body therapy and immunotherapy.

Result: Total remission of all lung metastases within two years. No sign of detectable cancer up to patient's death at age 69 years from heart attack.

Case history No. 183/53:
Mrs. E. D. (born October 4th, 1898)

TOTAL REMISSION OF PRIMARY INOPERABLE UTERINE CANCER

October 1952: Primary inoperable utero-cervical cancer, stage III, infiltrating the total right side parametrium space on to pelvic wall. Remission after radiotherapy.

March 1953: First relapse. Patient refuses further radiation. Progression of tumour in subsequent six months. Then admission to Issels-Klinik.

Condition on admission, September 1953:
Terminal stage. The minor pelvic space totally walled up by solid tumour. Impossible to palpate extent of tumour.

Treatment: Whole-body therapy and immunotherapy.

Result: Complete disappearance of all malignant symptoms. For further twenty years no signs of detectable cancer.

Case history No. 49/54:

Mrs. J. K. (born February 7th, 1914)

TOTAL REMISSION OF INCURABLE OVARIAN CARCIN-OMA

August 1953: Laparotomy reveals existence of incurable bilaterial ovarian neoplasia with multiocular carcinomatous disseminations with concomitant sanguinolent ascites. Histopathology: Cyst-Adeno-Carcinoma of both ovaries.

September 1953: Sub-total resection of all reachable tumour masses, total hysterectomy and bilateral salpingo-oophorectomy. Intra-abdominal instillation of radio-gold. Follow-up radiotherapy, no regression, only progression. Prognosis hopeless. Patient referred to the Issels-Klinik.

Condition on admission, January 26th, 1954:
Vaginal examination reveals sizable tumours.

Treatment: Whole-body therapy and immunotherapy.

Result: Regression of all tumours. No signs of detectable cancer until last contact in 1963.

Case history No. 56/55:

Mr. K. H. K. (born March 9th, 1925)

TOTAL REMISSION OF GENERALISED METASTASES FOLLOWING SURGERY OF SEMINOMA

December 1954: right-sided testicle eradicated by surgery. Histopathology: Seminoma. Postoperative radiation recommended because of several palpable lymphnodes on the right side. Patient refused. Admitted to the Issels-Klinik.

Condition on admission, January 1955:
Induration within the cicatrice area of the right-side groin. In the following months: swelling of the left testicle, concomitant inguinal lymphomata. Development of a syndrome characterising metastatic lesion in the pubic bone and left-side epigastric space.

Treatment: Whole-body therapy and immunotherapy.

Result: Total remission of all tumour symptoms. The patient subsequently married and fathered two children. No further signs of detectable cancer in the following nineteen years.

Case history No. 257/55:
Mr. E. B. (born March 5th, 1911)

TOTAL REMISSION OF RECURRING SARCOMATA OF SOFT PARTS

February 1955: Several neoplasia of soft parts of thighs removed by surgery. Histopathology: Large-cellular-round-cell sarcoma. No follow-up treatment.

September 1955: First recurrence appeared on left-sided shank. No surgery or radiotherapy. Patient admitted to the Issels-Klinik.

Condition on admission, October 1955:
Infiltration of the left-sided lower leg.

Treatment: Whole-body therapy and immunotherapy.

Result: Complete remission.

July 1957: Second recurrence on left-sided lower leg. Immediate re-admission to the Issels-Klinik.

Result: Total remission without any relapse for the following sixteen years.

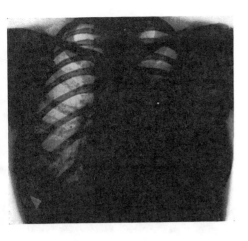 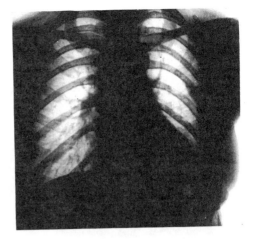

Before whole-body therapy   15 years later

Case history No 166/52
Total remission of recurring pleural sarcoma

Case history No 98/56
Total remission of a thyroid carcinoma

Before whole-body therapy   4 months later

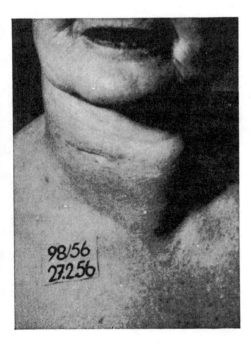 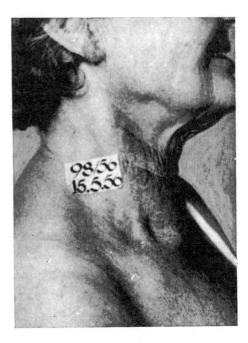

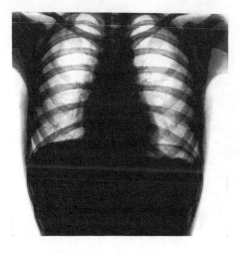

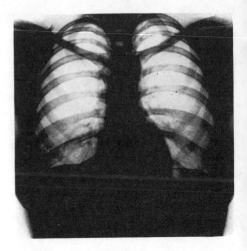

Before whole-body therapy   14½ years later

Case history No 233/56
Total remission of a recurring lymphosarcoma

Case history No 171/66
Total remission of an incurable pulmonary sarcoma

Before whole-body therapy   4½ years later

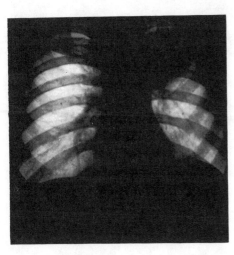

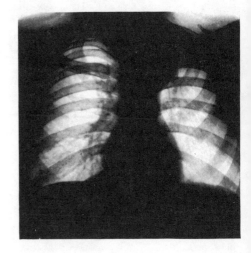

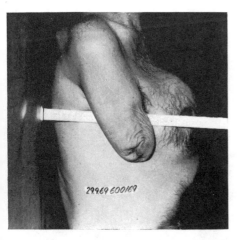 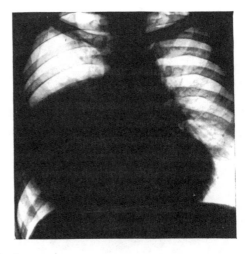

Before whole-body therapy

Case history No 600/69
Total remission of a mediastinal teratoma

7 months later

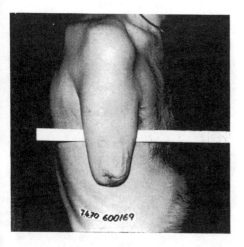 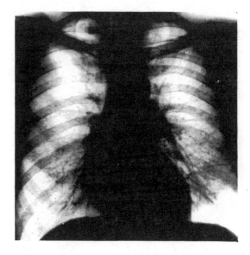

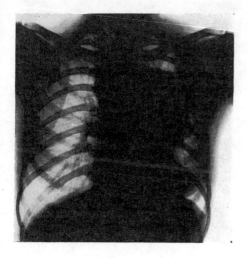 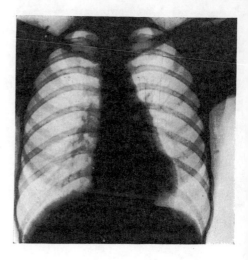

Before whole-body therapy   10 months later

Case history No 10325/72
Total remission of a non-treated Morbus Hodgkin

Case history No 160/54
Total remission of an untreated bronchus cancer

Before whole-body therapy   14½ years later

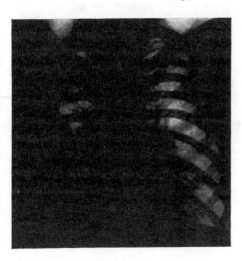 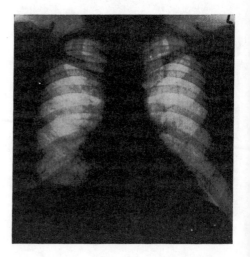

Case history No. 76/56:
Mrs. H. S. (born March 9th, 1933)

TOTAL REMISSION OF A RECURRING CEREBELLAR TUMOUR

October 1948: Surgical eradication and follow-up radiotherapy of a brain tumour. Histopathology: Cerebellar Astrocytoma.

October 1955: Second operation because of recurring cerebellar tumour. Histopathology: Spongioblastoma. Palliative sub-total surgery. Patient refuses urgently advised radiotherapy. Three months later with progressive symptoms admitted to Issels-Klinik. Prognosis hopeless.

Condition on admission, January 1956:
Cranial nerves outfall-syndrome due to neoplastic cerebral tumour.

Treatment: Whole-body therapy and immunotherapy.

Result: Total regression of all tumour symptoms. No further signs of detectable cancer in the subsequent eighteen years.

Case history No. 98/56:

Mrs. G.-L. K. (born May 23rd, 1891)

TOTAL REMISSION OF A THYROID CARCINOMA

December 1955: A goiter verified by histological examination to be a struma maligna. Patient refuses urgently advised surgery and radio–therapy. Admitted to Issels-Klinik without any previous treatment.

Condition on admission, February 22nd, 1956:
Mainly right-sided thyroid tumour increasing the circumference of the neck to 37 cm. A large metastatic lymphgland is palpable and visible behind the left-sided mandibular angle.

Treatment: Whole-body therapy and immunotherapy.

Result: Total regression in three months. No signs of detectable cancer in the subsequent fourteen years until patient died at 80 from natural causes.

Case history No. 233/56:
Child U. H. (born March 12th, 1944)

TOTAL REMISSION OF RECURRING LYMPHOSARCOMA

April 1956: Examination reveals multiple small lymphomata, including a single egg-sized tumour rapidly growing in cervical region.
The mediastinal and hilar lymphnodes also increase. Histopathology:
Lymphosarcoma. Total regression of all detectable malignancy after
radio and chemotherapy. Six weeks later recurrence of all tumours;
mediastinal neoplasms reshape. Prognosis hopeless. Admission to
Issels-Klinik.

Condition on admission, July 1956:
Spreading of mediastinal and hilar formations, multiple small solid
lymphomata in both cervical regions.

Treatment: Whole-body therapy and immunotherapy.

Result: Total regression of all tumour symptoms. Patient married
and is mother of two healthy children. No signs of detectable cancer
for the past seventeen years.

Case history No. 304/56:

Mrs. Th. B. (born May 3rd, 1907)

TOTAL REMISSION OF INCURABLE UTERIN CANCER

October 1954: Utero-cervical neoplasia, stage II. Histopathology: Platy-cellular-carcinoma. Surgery performed.

January 1955: First recurrence. Regression after radiotherapy.

August 1956: Second recurrence. Malignant infiltration of the bladder. Obstruction of the right-sided ureter, nephro-hydrosis. Prognosis hopeless. Patient admitted to the Issels-Klinik.

Condition on admission, September 1956:
Infiltration between right-side of vaginal vault and pelvic wall.

Treatment: Whole-body therapy and immunotherapy.

Result: Total remission. Eighteen years have passed without any further signs of detectable cancer.

Case history No. 381/56:
Mrs. R.W. (born December 4th, 1928)

TOTAL REMISSION OF AN UNTREATED PRIMARY UTERINE CANCER

November 1956: Cancer of the uterus. Histopathology: Invasive Platy-cellular carcinoma. Patient refuses surgery and radiotherapy. Admitted to the Issels-Klinik without any previous treatment.

Condition on admission, January 1957:
Uterine induration infiltrating into the right-sided parametrium. In the following weeks progressive tumour growth until stage II.

Treatment: Whole-body therapy and immunotherapy.

Result: Total remission. Seventeen years have passed without any further signs of detectable cancer.

Case history No. 159/60:

Mrs. A. S. (born March 14th, 1909)

TOTAL REMISSION OF A PRIMARY INCURABLE BRAIN TUMOUR

November 1959: Surgical exploration reveals a wide-spread cerebral neoplasia, which has already demolished an area of the right-sided skullbase and totally walled up the orbital cavity and sphenoidal sinus of the same side. Histopathology: Duro-sarcoma.

The malignant tissues, as far as possible, are subtotally resected. The rather voluminous residual malignancies are subjected to follow-up radiotherapy. This palliative measure is unsuccessful because Duro-sarcoma is not radiosensitive. Prognosis hopeless. Patient admitted to Issels-Klinik.

Condition on admission, March 1960:
Very bad general condition, increasing brain pressure, hemicrania left side, ataxia.

Treatment: Whole-body therapy and immunotherapy.

Result: Complete remission within one year. No further signs of detectable cancer in the subsequent fourteen years.

Case history No. 171/66:

Mr. D. M. (born August 23rd, 1946)

TOTAL REMISSION OF AN INCURABLE PULMONARY SARCOMA

November 1965: Detection of a tumour in upper lobe bronchus of left-sided lung. Histopathology: Spindle-cell sarcoma. Radiotherapy with tele-cobalt, limited success. Then new development of tumour and hemorrhage. Prognosis hopeless. Admission to Issels-Klinik.

Condition on admission, March 1966:
Massive shadow in the right-sided superior pulmonal lobe.

Treatment: Whole-body therapy and immunotherapy, initially combined with small doses of chemotherapy.

Results: Total remission of the malignancy. No detectable signs of cancer in eight subsequent years.

Case history No. 406/67:

Mrs. A. C. (born January 6th, 1923)

TOTAL REMISSION OF A SUB-TOTALLY REMOVED META-STASISING SIGMOID CARCINOMA

April 1967: Surgical intervention revealed a metastasising sigmoidal neoplasm which already had infested the liver. Histopathology: Adeno-carcinoma.

May 1967: Sub-total resection performed. The intestinal primary tumour plus reachable para-aortal lymphomata removed. Liver metastases which showed progression since the first surgery remained untouched. Patient admitted to the Issels-Klinik. Prognosis hopeless.

Condition on admission, June 1967:
Hepatic metastases of a sigmoid carcinoma, twice verified by biopsy and scintigraphy.

Treatment: Whole-body therapy and immunotherapy.

Result: Total regression of all tumours. No detectable signs of cancer in seven subsequent years.

Case history No. 447/67:
Child G. P. (born June 21st, 1957)

TOTAL REMISSION OF RETICULAR SARCOMA

June 1967: Suspected neoplasia involving the fascia lata area of right-sided thigh. Histopathology: Reticular sarcoma. Radical femoral amputation and radiotherapy advised. Parents refused. Patient admitted to Issels-Klinik.

Condition on admission, July 1967:
X-Rays reveal infestation of femoral bone within a triangular area measuring 4 x 2 cm.

Treatment: Whole-body therapy and immunotherapy.

Result: Total regression of the malignancy. No detectable signs of cancer in seven subsequent years.

Case history No. 600/69:

Mr. K.W. (born April 28th, 1926)

TOTAL REMISSION OF A MEDIASTINAL TERATOMA

November 1964: Eradication of a mediastinal malignancy.
Histopathology: Teratoma. Follow-up radiation and chemotherapy.

October 1968: First relapse in the right-sided anterior mediastinal space. Further surgery and radiotherapy advised and refused by patient. Chemotherapy agents applied. They offer only limited help. Then rapid growth develops. Prognosis hopeless. Patient admitted to Issels-Klinik.

Condition on admission, August 1969:
Radiological examination shows a massive dense shadow on the lower right half of the pulmonal field. Immense tumour of the anterior chest wall measuring 15 cm x 27 cm.

Treatment: Whole-body therapy and immunotherapy, initially combined with two shots of Cyclo-phosphamide.

Result: Total remission of malignancy without any further relapse.

Case history No. 204/70:
Child J. G. (born March 21st, 1961)

TOTAL REMISSION OF A PRIMARY INCURABLE PELVIC SPACE TERATOMA

November 1969: Exploratory laparatomy reveals massive tumour in pelvic space. Inoperable, adherent to sacrum and rectum. Histopathology: Malignant teratoma. Following Betatron and Gammatron radiations show that the malignancy does not respond. Progressive tumour growth. Prognosis hopeless. Patient admitted to Issels-Klinik.

Condition on admission, February 1970:
Hypogastrium filled with neoplasma measuring 16 cm x 11 cm. Egg-sized metastasis in the left-sided inguinal area.

Treatment: Whole-body therapy and immunotherapy.

Result: Total remission of tumours without any further relapse.

Case history No. 784/70:

Child D. T. (born August 21st, 1965)

REGRESSION OF AN INCURABLE LYMPHO-SARCOMA

December 1968: A right-sided cervical lymphoma, originally identified as Morbus Hodgkin. Unsuccessful radiotherapy. Renewed biopsy. Histopathology: Lympho-sarcoma in August 1969. Chemotherapy halted because of patient's incompatibility to treatment. Prognosis hopeless. Patient admitted to Issels-Klinik.

Condition on admission, November 1970:
Right-sided neck: two chestnut-sized lymphomata. Smaller lymphomata in both groins.

Treatment: Whole-body therapy and immunotherapy.

Result: Total regression of all tumour symptoms.

November 1971: Relapse. Progressive osteolytic destruction in the anteror skull-base with concomitant hydrocephalus.

Treatment: Whole-body therapy and immunotherapy with additional chemotherapy during the first two months.

Result: Total remission of all tumour symptoms including intracranial involvement. There has been no subsequent relapse.

Case history No. 10325/72:
Miss M. H. (born December 7th, 1952)

TOTAL REMISSION OF A NON-TREATED MORBUS HODGKIN STAGE III

February 1972: Cervical lymphomata. Histopathology: Morbus Hodgkin. Clinical stage III. Surgery impossible. Radiotherapy advised and refused. Admission to Issels-Klinik.

Condition on admission, April 1972:
In the left-sided cervical region as well as in the region between the left-sided mamma and armpit multiple lymphomata. Retro-abdominal tumours palpable. Massive left-sided hilar shadow.

Treatment: Whole-body therapy and immunotherapy initially combined with small doses of chemotherapy.

Result: Total remission of all tumour signs and symptoms without any further relapse.

Case history No. 160/54:

Mr. H. K. (born March 29th, 1910)

TOTAL REMISSION OF AN UNTREATED BRONCHUS CANCER

June 1954: Tomographic pulmonary radiographs reveal stenosis of the right-sided main bronchus with arrosion of the bronchial wall and concomitant carcinomatous infiltration of the per-bronchial space. Surgery and radiation advised and refused. Admission to Issels-Klinik with hopeless prognosis.

Condition on admission, July 1954:

Large shadow in the right-sided inferior pulmonal space originating from the right hilus and adherent to the diaphragm.

Treatment: Whole-body therapy and immunotherapy.

Result: Total remission of all tumour signs. No detectable cancer in the subsequent twenty years.

Bibliography

Bibliography

van AAKEN, E.: 'Statistischer Beweis einer möglichen Krebs-Prophylaxe ...' Dr. E. van Aaken, 4056 Schwalmtal-Waldniel (Niederrh.) 1971

ABDERHALDEN, E.: *Abwehrfermente*. Th. Steinkopff, Dresden u. Leipzig. 6. Aufl. 1941

ABDERHALDEN, E.: 'Studien über die Verwendbarkeit der Abwehr-Proteinase-Reaktion zur Diagnose des Carcinoms'. *Schweiz. Med. Wschr.* 76 (1946) S. 47

ABEL, W.: 'Statistisches zum Krebsproblem'. *Z. Krebsforsch.* 56 (1948/50) Nr. 1, S. 36–79

ABRAMS, G. D. et al.: 'Influence of the Normal Flora on Mucosal Morphology and Cellular Renewal in the Ileum'. *Laborat. Investigation* (USA) 1963 (12. März)

ACKERKNECHT, E. H.: *Geschichte und Geographie der wichtigsten Krankheiten*. F. Enke, Stuttgart 1963

ACKERMANN, G.: 'Immuntherapeutische Probleme'. *Prophylaxe 8* (1969) Nr. 8, S. 176–183

ADAM, W.: 'Zum Thema: Die barmherzige Lüge'. *Medizinische* (1959) Nr. 25, S. 1185–1189

ADAMKIEWICZ, A.: *Untersuchungen über den Krebs und das Prinzip seiner Behandlung*. W. Braumüller, Leipzig-Wien 1893

ALEXANDER, P.: 'Immunotherapy of leukemia: The use of different classes of immune lymphocytes'. *Cancer Res.* 27 (1967) 2512

ALTMANN, L.: 'Propädeutik der Herdlehre ...' *Jahresberichte* d. DAH 15 (1967/68) S. 109–114

ANDERSON, M. R. u. GREEN, H. N.: 'Tumour Host Relationships'. *Brit. J. Cancer* 21 (1967) Nr. 1, S. 27–32

ANEMUELLER, H. u. RIES, J.: 'Anleitung zu einer stoffwechsel-aktiven Kost'. *Bayer. Krebsges. e. V.*, München 1970 von ARDENNE, M.: 'Theoretische und experimentelle Grundlagen der Krebs-Mehrschritt-Therapie'. VEB *Verlag Volk u. Gesundheit*, Berlin-Jena. 2. Aufl. 1970/71

ARMSTRONG, D., SOMERSON, G. u. HAYFLICK, L.: Cytopathogenic Mycoplasmas Associated with two human tumors'. *J. Bact.* 90 (1965) S. 418

ASCHOFF, L.: Rudolf VIRCHOW (Geistiges Europa-Bändchen). Hoffmann u. Campe, Hamburg. 2. Aufl. 1948

ASCHNER, B.: 'Ist die Unterdrückung der Hämorrhoidal- und Menstrualblutungen belanglos?' *Münch. Med. Wschr.* 1934, Nr. 12

ASCHNER, B.: *Befreiung der Medizin vom Dogma.* K. F. Haug 1962

AUDIER, A. G.: 'Immunotherapie metastasierender Malignome'. *Medizinische 1959*, Nr. 40, S. 1860–1864

AULER, H.: *Über Wartung und Behandlung Krebskranker.* München 1935

AULER, H.: 'Über die zusätzliche Behandlung Krebskranker'. *Z. Krebsforsch.* 47 (1938) S. 126

BAHNSON, C. B. et al.: 'Die Bedeutung des eigenen Abwehrvermögens bei der Ätiologie maligner Tumoren'. Ann. N.Y. Acad. Sc. 125 (1966) S. 827. – Ref. in: *Krebsarzt 22* (1967) S. 48

BAILEY, H.: *Krebiozen – Key to Cancer?* Hermitage House, New York, N.Y. 1955

BARTH, G., HUTH, E. u. WACHSMANN, F.: 'Experimentelle Untersuchungen zur Frage der Hyperthermie bösartiger Geschwülste'. *Strahlentherapie* 88 (1952) S. 1

BAUER, K. H.: *Das Krebsproblem.* Springer, Berlin-Göttingen-Heidelberg. 1. Aufl. 1949, 2. Aufl. 1963

BAZALA, W.: 'Wie weit sind wir in der Krebsfrage vorgedrungen?' *Ars Medici* 1959, Nr. 9, S. 611–625

BECKER, A.: *Der Krebs der Menschen.* Orell Füssli, Zürich 1935

BEGEMANN, H.: 'Das Blut als Organ'. In.: BÜCHNER-LETTERER-ROULER: *Handb. d. Allg. Pathologie.* Band III/2, S. 1–43. Springer, Berlin 1960

BENKÖ, A., KOLTAY, M. u. GABOR, P.: 'Über die Fernwirkung karzinogener Stoffe mit besonderer Berücksichtigung der Leberveränderungen'. Arch. f. Geschwulstforsch. 5 (1953) S. 47

BERGUT, F. A.: 'Der Zustand des Blutgerinnungssystems bei Krebskranken'. *Sowjetsk. Med.* 1967, Nr. 5, S. 102. – Ref. in: *Krebsarzt* 23 (1968) S. 114

BINGOLD, K.: 'Die Behandlung unheilbarer Krankheitszustände . . .'
Med. Klin. 50 (1955) S. 22

BIRCHER-BENNER, M.: *Ernährungskrankheiten.* Wendepunkt-
Verlag, Zürich 1943

BITTNER, J. J.: 'The Causes and Control of Mammary Cancer in
Mice'. (Vortrag i. d. HARVEY-Ges. am 20.2.1947) *Krebsarzt* 3
(1948) Nr. 9, S. 321

BORREL, A.: 'Évolution cellulaire et parasitisme dans l'épithélioma'.
– Thèse. Montpellier 1892

BORST, M.: *Die Lehre von den Geschwülsten.* 2 Bände. J. F. Bergmann,
Wiesbaden. 1. Aufl. 1902

BOSHAMER, K. u. KOCH, F. W.: 'Versuch, die Reaktion auf
Carcinom-Extrakt-Injektion diagnostisch auszuwerten'. *Z. Krebs-*
forsch. 57 (1950) S. 339–342

BRAUNSTEIN, A.: 'Über immunologische Krebsprophylaxe und
konstitutionelle Krebsdisposition'. *Z. Krebsforsch.* 39 (1933) S. 321

von BREHMER, W.: 'Krebs – eine Erregerkrankheit'. *Fortschr. Med.*
1932, Nr. 17, S. 50

BRÜDA, B. E.: 'Die Bedeutung des R-E-S für das Blastom-
Wachstum'. *Z. Krebsforsch.* 34 (1931) S. 185

BURGKHARDT, F.: 'Die zusätzliche biologische Behandlung des
Krebses mit hochwertigen Coli-Stämmen (Mutaflor) und Leber-
Extrakten'. *Mschr. f. Krebsbekämpf.* 9 (1941) S. 97

BURNET: *Immunological Surveillance.* Pergamon Press, Oxford 1970

BUSSE-GRAWITZ, P.: *Experimentelle Grundlagen zu einer modernen*
Pathologie. B. Schwabe & Co, Basel 1946

BUTTERSACK, F.: *Latente Erkrankungen des Grundgewebes.* Stuttgart
1912

CAUM, S.: *Cancer Cures Crucified.* Caumsette Press, Drexel Hill,
Penn. 1968

CHIURCO. G. A.: 'Neue Gesichtspunkte zur Präcancerogenese'.
Z. Blut- und Geschwulst-Krankh. 2 (1970) Nr. 3, S. 49–54

CHRISTIANI, A.: 'Die Aufklärung der FREUND-NEUBERG-schen
cytolytischen Phänomene führt zu neuen Überlegungen hinsichtlich
der Abwehrreaktionen gegen Krebs'. *Österr. Z. Krebsforsch.* (früher:
Krebsarzt) 26 (1971) Nr. 4, S. 255–263

COHNHEIM, J.: *Vorlesungen über Allgemeine Pathologie.* Berlin, 1. Aufl.
1875, 2. Aufl. 1882

CRAMER, H. u. GUMMEL, H.: 'Richtlinien für die Früherkennung, Behandlung und Vorbeugung von bösartigen Geschwülsten'. *Strahlentherapie* 85, Nr. 3 u. Deutscher Ärztekalender 1954, S. 346–355

CRILE, G., SCHOFIELD, P. F.: 'Effect of Lymphatic Obstruction on the Growth and Metastasis of Tumors'. *Surg. Gynaec. Obstet.* 128 (1969) S. 1042

CURRY, M.: *Biolimatik.* 2 Bände. Bioclimatic Research Institute. Riederau/Ammersee 1946

DEMMER, F.: 'Über Krebsoperationen, deren Vor- und Nachbehandlung, besonders beim Mammakarzinom'. *Krebsarzt* 1 (1946) Nr. 7, S. 271–294

DEMMER, F.: 'Zur Radikaloperation des Mammakarzinoms und über die eingeschränkte Radikaloperation'. *Krebsarzt* 9 (1945) Nr. 2, S. 65–82

DIEHL, J. C. u. TROMP, S. W.: *Probleme der geographischen Häufigkeitsverteilung der Krebssterblichkeit in Holland.* K. F. Haug, Ulm 1955

DOMAGK, G.: 'Welche Erkenntnisse über Krebs vermittelt uns die experimentelle Krebsforschung?' *Münch. Med. Wschr.* 94 (1952) Nr. 37, S. 1841

DOMAGK, G.: 'Die Entwicklung der Carcinom-Therapie. (Vortrag auf d. Dtsch. Therapiewoche, Karlsruhe 1954) *Ärztl. Praxis* 6 (1954) Nr. 36

DOSCH, P.: 'Krebsgeschehen und Neuraltherapie'. *Erfahrungsheilk.* 20 (1971) Nr. 3, S. 65–72

DOSCH, P.: *Lehrbuch der Neuraltherapie nach HUNEKE.* K. F. Haug, Heidelberg. 3. Aufl. 1971

DRUCKREY, H.: 'Die Grundlagen der Krebsentstehung'. In: *Grundlagen und Praxis chemischer Tumorbehandlung.* Springer, Berlin 1954

DRUCKREY, H.: 'Krebserzeugende Eigenschaften bei Arzneimitteln'. *Münch. Med. Wschr.* 98 (1956) Nr. 9, S. 295–297

EGER, W., JUNGMICHEL, H. u. TERRUHN, Ch.: 'Über Resistenzänderungen des Organismus und die Möglichkeit ihrer Beeinflussung'. *Medizinische* 1958, S. 605

EHRICH, W. E. 'Die Entzündung'. In BÜCHNER-LETTERER-ROULET: *Handbuch der Allg. Pathologie,* J. Springer, Berlin 1956.

ENDERLEIN, G.: *Bakterien-Cyklogenie.* Walter de Gruyter & Co, Berlin 1925

EPPINGER, H.: *Permeabilitäts-Pathologie*. Springer, Wien 1949

FARRENSTEINER, E. u. FARRENSTEINER, Ch.: *Blutdiagonstik im Dunkelfeld*. Farrensteiner, Bad Salzdetfurth 1969

FEYRTER, F.: 'Über die Pathologie peripherer vegetativer Regulationen ...' In: BÜCHNER-LETTERER-ROULET: *Handb. d. Allg. Pathologie*. Band VIII/2, S. 344. Springer, Berlin 1966

FISCHER, W.: 'Die Reaktion des Organismus bei bösartigen Geschwülsten'. *Wiss. Zschr. d. Univ. Jena* 1951/52, Nr. 3

FISCHER-WASELS, B.: 'Allgemeine Geschwulstlehre'. In: BETHE-BERGMANN-EMBDEN-ELLINGER: *Handb. der normalen u. pathologischen Physiologie*. Band XIV/2. Springer, Berlin 1927

FISCHER-WASELS, B.: *Wege zur Verhütung der Entstehung und Ausbreitung der Krebskrankheit*. Springer, Berlin 1934

FISCHER-WASLES, B.: 'Die Bedeutung der besonderen Allgemeindisposition des Körpers für die Entstehung der Krebskrankheit und die Möglichkeit ihrer Bekämpfung'. *Strahlentherapie* 50 (1935) S. 5

FLEISCHHACKER, H.:' Zur klinischen Bedeutung des Herdgeschehens'. *Österr. Z. Stomat.* 60 (1963) S. 10

FREUND, E.: 'Die Bakterienflora des Darmes und maligne Tumoren'. *Krebsarzt* 2 (1947) S. 382–386

FREUND, E. u. KAMINER, G.: *Biochemische Grundlagen der Disposition für Carcinom*. Springer, Berlin u. Wien 1925

FROMME, A.: *Das Mesenchym und die Mesenchym-Theorie des Karzinoms*. Th. Steinkopff, Dresden u. Leipzig 1953

FUDALLA, S. G.: 'Der kranke Zahn als Mesenchymstörer'. *Erfahrungsheilk.* 15 (1966) Nr. 12, S. 376–383

FUDALLA, S. G.: 'Symbiologie als Ganzheitsschau', *Phys. Med. u. Rehabil.* 9 (1968) Nr. 12, S. 333–336

GÄBELEIN, K.: 'Zur Frage der Existenz der Thioäther beim gangränosen Abbau'. *Dtsch. Zahnärztl. Zeitschr.* 15 (1960) Nr. 10, S. 806–808

GASCHLER, A.: 'Fermente und Krebs'. *Hippokrates* 28 (1957) Nr. 3

GERICKE, D., SCHÜTZE, E.: 'Versuche zur Beeinflussung des Tumorwachstums durch Mykoplasmen'. *Zbl. Bakt.*, I. Abt. Orig. 210 (1969) S. 212

GERLACH, F.: *Krebs und obligater Pilzparasitismus*. Urban & Schwarzenberg, Wien 1948

GERLACH, F.: 'Über Auffindung, Benennung und Beurteilung von in malignen Tumoren aufgefundenen Mikroorganismen'. *Krebsarzt* 6 (1951) Nr. 3/4, S. 86

GERLACH, F.: 'Immunbiologische Studien bei malignen Tumoren und Haemoblastosen. *Krebsarzt* 16 (1961) Nr. 2, S. 54

GERSON, M.: *A Cancer Therapy*. Dura Books, New York, N.Y. 1958

GLASER-TÜRK, M.: 'Die modernen experimentellen Grundlagenerkenntnisse des Herdgeschehens'. *Fortbildungshefte d. Internat. Ges. f. Elektroakupunktur e. V.*, Juli 1971, Nr. 1

GLEMSER, B.: *Man Against Cancer*. The Bodley Head Ltd., London 1969

GOLDBLATT, H. u. CAMERON, G.: 'Induced Malignancy in Cells from Rat Myocardium Subjected to Intermittent Anaërobiosis during Long Propagation In Vitro'. *J. of Exper. Med.* 97/11 (1953) S. 525

GOOD, R. A. u. GABRIELSEN, A. E.: *The Thymus in Immunobiology*. Hoeber/New York u. Evanston/London 1964

GRAF, H.: 'Das Problem der körpereigenen Abwehr beim Krebswachstum'. Dr. A. Hüthig, Heidelberg 1969

GRAFF, S., MOORE, D. H., STANLEY, W. M., RANDALL, H. T. u. HAGENSEN, C. D.: 'Isolation of Mouse Mammary Carcinoma-Virus'. *Cancer* 2 (1949) Nr. 5, S. 755

GRAFFI, A.: 'Beitrag zur Wirkungsweise cancerogener Reize und zur Frage des chemischen Aufbaus normaler und maligner Zellen'. *Arch. f. Geschwulstforsch.* 1 (1949) Nr. 1/2 S. 61–121

GRAFFI, A.: 'Virusarten als Geschwulstursache'. *Ars Medici* 59 (1969) Nr. 7, S. 447–468

GRAFFI, A., HEBEKERL, W. et al.: 'Über chemische Frühveränderungen der Rattenleber nach Vertfütterung cancerogener Azo-Farbstoffe'. *Arch. f. Geschwulstforsch.* 5 (1953) Nr. 1, S. 1–24 u. Nr. 2, S. 101–110

GREEN, H. N.: 'Immunological Aspects of Cancer'. In: WOLSTENHOLME, G. E. u. O'CONNOR, M.: *Ciba Foundation Symposion on Carcinogenesis*. J. u. A. Churchill, London 1959

GREEN, H. N. et al.: *An Immunological Approach to Cancer*. Butterworths, London 1967. – Ref. in: *Krebsarzt* 24 (1969) S. 261

GREENE, W. A. et al.: 'Psychological Factors and Reticulo-Endothelial Disease'. *Psychosomat. Med.* 16 (1954) S. 220–230 u. 18 (1956) S. 284–303

GROTE, L. R.: 'Die seelische Führung des krebskranken Menschen'. *Therapiewoche* 5 (1954) S. 11–16

GRUNDMANN, E.: 'Cancerogenese aus molekularer Sicht'. Vortrag auf dem 17. Internat. Fortbildungskongreß, Davos 1969. – Ref. in: *Dtsch. Ärztblatt* 1969, Nr. 38, S. 2613–2616

GÜNTHER, O.: *Einführung in die Imunbiologie.* Hippokrates-Verlag, Stuttgart 1969

HACKMANN, Ch.: 'Die Bedeutung einer ... Resistenz-Steigerung ... für das Tumorwachstum'. Vortrag auf der Arbeitstagung d. 'Ges. z. Bekämpf. d. Krebskrankh., Nordrhein-Westfalen e. V.', Dez. 1962

HAEHL, R.: *Samuel HAHNEMANN* – sein Leben und Werk. 2 Bände. 1922

HALL, J. G. u. SMITH, M. E.: 'Homing of Lymph-Borne Immunoblasts to the Gut'. *Nature* 226 (1970) S. 262–263

HARRIS, R. J. C. (Ed.): *What We Know About Cancer.* George Allen & Unwin Ltd., London 1970

HARTMANN, E.: *Krankheit als Standortproblem.* K. F. Haug. Heidelberg, 2. Aufl. 1967

HEITAN, H.: 'Erfahrungen mit dem Mikrocolor-Test bei Krebskranken'. *Ärztl. Laborat.* 5 (1959) Nr. 2, S. 54–57

HELLSTRÖM, K. E. u. HELLSTRÖM, I.: 'Einige Aspekte der zellulären und der humoralen Immunreaktion auf Tumorantigene'. *Triangel* (Sandoz) 11 (1972) S. 23–28

HENSCHEN, C.: 'Die Behandlung des Carcinoms in der Chirurgie'. *Schweiz. Med. Wschr.* 61 (1931) Nr. 19, S. 441–456

HERBERGER, W.: *Behandlung und Pflege inoperabler Geschwulstkranker.* Th. Steinkopff, Dresden u. Leipzig 1960

HESS, M. W.: 'Lymphatischer Apparat, insbesondere Thymus, in der Pathogenese der Defekt-Immunopathien'. In: BÜCHNER-LETTERER-ROULET: *Handb. d. Allg. Pathologie.* Band VII/3, S. 182–236. Springer, Berlin 1970

HILLER: *Herderkrankungen, Grundlagenforschung u. Praxis.* C. Hanser, München 1956

HINSBERG, K.: *Das Geschwulstproblem in Chemie u. Physiologie.* Th. Steinkopff, Dresden u. Leipzig 1942

HINSBERG: 'Laboratoriumsmethoden zum Nachweis der Geschwulsterkrankungen'. Vortrag auf dem 5. Berchtesgadener Kurs für Ganzheitsmedizin. – Ref. in ZABEL, W.: *Ganzheitsbehandlung der Geschwulsterkrankungen.* Hippokrates-Verlag, Stuttgart 1953

208

HOFF, F.: *Klinische Physiologie und Pathologie*. G. Thieme, Stuttgart 1954

HOFF, F.: *Fieber. Unspezifische Abwehrvorgänge. Unspezifische Therapie*. G. Thieme, Stuttgart 1957

HOFFMANN, M.: 'Die Wirkung lokaler Überwärmungsmaßnahmen auf das Jensen-Sarkom und auf das Walker-Karzinom der Ratten'. *Arch. f. Geschwulstforsch.* 6 (1954) Nr. 2, S. 186–192

HOLDER, E., MEYTHALER, F., du MESNIL de ROCHEMONT, R. (Hrsg.): *Therapie maligner Tumoren, Hämoblastome und Hämoblastosen.* 3 Bände. F. Enke, Stuttgart 1966–1968–1969

HOLLOS, J.: *Immune-Blood Therapy of Tuberculosis.* New York 1938

HUMPHREY, J. H. u. WHITE, R. G.: *Kurzes Lehrbuch der Immunologie.* G. Thieme, Stuttgart 1971

HUNEKE, F.: *Das Sekundenphänomen.* K. F. Haug, Ulm-Heidelberg 1965

HUTH, E.: 'Die Rolle der bakteriellen Infektionen bei der Spontanremission maligner Tumoren und Leukosen'. In: LAMPERT-SELAWRY: *Körpereigene Abwehr und bösartige Geschwülste.* K. F. Haug, Ulm 1957

ISSELS, J.: *Grundlagen und Richtlinien für eine Interne Krebstherapie.* Hippokrates-Verlag, Stuttgart 1953

ISSELS, J.: 'Ergebnisse und Erkenntnisse nach vierjähriger klinisch-interner Therapie beim inkurablen Krebskranken'. *Hipokrates 25* (1954) Nr. 16, S. 514–529 (u. Bildbeilage)

ISSELS, J.: 'Karzinom – aus dem Blut-Eiweißbild ablsebar?' *Med. Mschr.* 1955, Nr. 11, S. 755–756

ISSELS, J.: 'Gedanken zur internen Behandlung von Tumorkranken'. *Hippokrates 27* (1956) Nr. 6, S. 173–180 (u. Bildbeilage)

ISSELS, J.: 'Fokalinfekt und Krebs'. *Dtsch. Zahnärztl. Zeitschr.* 11 (1956) Nr. 3, S. 123–131

ISSELS, J.: 'Können wurzelbehandelte Zähne Krebs erzeugen?' *Das Dtsch. Zahnärzteblatt* 1956, Nr. 19

ISSELS, J.: 'Die Rolle des Herdes im Rahmen der internen Geschwulstbehandlung'. *Therapiewoche 9* (1958/59) Nr. 2

ISSELS, J. u. WINSTOSSER, K.: 'Ganzheitliche interne Krebstherapie'. *Erfahrungsheilk.* 17 (1968) Nr. 11 u. 12

ISSELS, J.: *Die Ernährung des Krebskranken und Krebsgefährdeten.* Sensen-Verlag, Wien 1970

ISSELS, J.: 'Stellungnahme zum Report der britischen Ärztekommission über die Therapie der Ringberg-Klinik'. *Krebsgeschehen* 1 (3) (1971) Nr. 1 (2), S. 25 (53) – 76 (104)

ISSELS, J.: *Über die Interne Krebsbehandlung in der Ringberg-Klinik. – Entgegnung auf den Bericht der britischen Ärztegruppe.* – Helfer-Verlag E. Schwabe, Bad Homburg v.d.H. 1971

ISSELS, J.: 'Die Nachbehandlung von Krebskranken'. *Gesundheitspolitische Umschau* 23 (1972) Nr. 4, S. 76

ISSELS, J.: *Mehr Heilungen von Krebs.* Helfer-Verlag E. Schwabe, Bad Homburg v.d.H. 1972

JACOB, F. u. MONOD, J.: 'Genetic Regulatory Mechanisms in the Synthesis of Proteins'. *J.Mol. Biol.* 3 (1961) S. 318–356

JOACHIM, H.: *Papyrus EBERS, das älteste Buch über Heilkunde.* Berlin 1890

JUNG, H.: *Krebs und Lebenshaltung im Lichte der Zellatmung.* Werk-Verlag Dr. E. Banaschewski, München-Gräfelfing 1957

KALLENBACH, H.: 'Beeinflussung der Metastasen-Häufigkeit durch Resistenz-Minderung'. *Langenbeck's Archiv. f. Klin. Chir. 300* (1962) S. 437–462

KALLENBACH, H.: 'Minderung der natürlichen Krebsabwehr durch Zytostatika?' *Med. Klin.* 59 (1964) S. 140

KAUFMANN, W.: 'Standortfaktoren und Krebsentstehung'. *Erfahrungsheilk.* 15 (1966) Nr. 4, S. 115–117

KELLNER, G.: 'Die Wirkung des Herdes auf die Labilität des humoralen Systems'. *Österr. Z. Stomat.* 60 (1963) S. 312

KLEIN, E. u. KLEIN, G.: 'Tumorantigene und ihre mögliche Anwendung in Forschung, Tumortherapie und Tumorprophylaxe'. *Triangel* (Sandoz) 11 (1972) S. 15–22

KNOLLE, G.: 'Gebißbefunde bei Tumorkranken zu Beginn der Nachkuren'. *Zahnärztl. Prax.* 16 (1965) Nr. 4, S. 37–38

KOLISKO, L.: Zit. aus WENDEL, K.: 'Anthroposophische Medizin und Homöopathie'. *Dtsch. Homöop. Mschr.* 4 (1953) Nr. 11, S. 519–524

KOLLATH, W.: 'Über die Mesotrophie, ihre Ursachen und praktische Bedeutung'. *Schriftenreihe d. Ganzheitsmedizin,* Band 3. Hippokrates-Verlag, Stuttgart

KOLLATH, W.: 'Versuche, betr. die Existenz der Siphonospora polymorpha v. BR'. *Hippokrates* 22 (1951) Nr. 4, S. 102–105

KOLLATH, W.: 'Dysbakterie, Tumorentstehung, Verhütung und Behandlung. Vortrag auf dem 5. Berchtesgadener Kurs für Ganzheitsmedizin'. – Ref. in: ZABEL, W.: *Ganzheitsbehandlung der Geschwulsterkrankungen.* Hippokrates-Verlag, Stuttgart 1953

KOLLATH, W.: *Die Ernährung als Naturwissenschaft.* K. F. Haug, Heidelberg 1967

KRAMER, F., THOMSEN, J. u. VOLL, R.: *Histologische, bakteriologische, statistische u. kasuistische Beiträge zum odontogenen Herdgeschehen.* Med. – Lit. Verlag Dr. Blume & Co, Uelzen

KRETZ, J.: 'Das Krebsleiden als Allgemeinerkrankung'. *Z. Krebsforsch.* 51 (1941) S. 6

KRETZ, J. u. PÖTZEL, O.: 'Die Psyche der Krebskranken'. *Krebsarzt* 1 (1946) S. 19

KRULL, P., LINDEMANN, F. W. u. KUNITSCH, G.: 'Dem Todkranken die Wahrheit sagen? (Zum Problem des offenen Gesprächs am Krankenbett)'. *Dtsch. Ärzteblatt* 69 (1972) Nr. 21, S. 1373–1375

LAMPERT, H.: *Heilung durch Überwärmung.* B. Wilkens, Hannover

LAMPERT, H. u. SELAWRY, O.: *Körpereigene Abwehr und bösartige Geschwülste.* K. F. Haug, Ulm 1957

LANG, N.: 'Immunologie des Carcinoms als Grundlage therapeutischer Überlegungen'. *Med. Welt* 1963, S. 2538

LETTRÉ, H.: 'Mitosegifte und cancerogene Faktoren als Antibiotika'. *Z. Krebsforsch.* 56 (1948) Nr. 1, S. 5–36

LICKINT, F.: *Zigarette und Lungenkrebs.* Hamm 1957 (Ferner: *Krebsforsch. u. Krebsbekämpfung* 3 (1959) S. 211)

LIEK, E.: *Krebsverbreitung, Krebsbekämpfung, Krebsverhütung.* J. F. Lehmann, München 1932

LINKE, A.: *Früherkennung des Krebses.* F. K. Schattauer, Stuttgart 1962

LIVINGSTON, V. W. – C.: *Cancer – A New Breakthrough.* Nash Publishing Corp., Los Angeles 1972

LOECKLE, W. E.: 'Seelisch-geistige Faktoren bei Krebs'. *Krebsarzt* 16 (1961) S. 207–216

LOECKLE, W E.: 'Das Massenexperiment am krebskranken Menschen'. (Heilziffern und echte Heilung) – *Heilkunde-Heilwege* 14 (1964) Nr. 4, S. 80–82

LUCKEY, Th. D.: *Germfree Life and Gnotobiology.* Academic Press, New York – London 1963

MAHNERT, A. u. MOSER, H.: 'Die Bedeutung funktioneller Störungen im Mesenchym für das Krankheitsgeschehen beim Krebs'. *Krebarzt* 5 (1950) S. 272–281

MATHÉ, G. et al.: *Presse Médicale* 74 (1966) S. 2615 u. *Rev. Franc. Étud. Clin. Biol.* 13 (1968) S. 454. – Zit. u.a.bei KREPLER, P.: *Krebsarzt* 24 (1969) Nr. 4, S. 208–220

MATHÉ, G.: *Méd. et Hyg.* (Frankr.) 29 (1971) S. 23. – Ref. in: *Selecta* 13 (1971) Nr. 47, S. 3775–3779 (Logistik in der Krebsbehandlung: Immuntherapie zusammen mit Chirurgie, Strahlen, Cytostatika'.)

MEYER, W.: 'Die anatomischen Grundlagen der Wurzelbehandlung'. *Dtsch. Zahnärztl. Zeitschr.* 15 (1960) Nr. 10, S. 777–786

MEYTHALER, F. u. HÄNDEL, F.: 'Zur Behandlung inoperabler Tumoren'. *Münch. Med. Wschr.* 94 (1952) Nr. 51, S. 2561–2570

MEYTHALER, F.u. TRUCKENBRODT, H.: 'Körpereigene Abwehr und Krebs'. *Ärztl. Prax.* 15 (1963) Nr. 1 u. 2

MIKHAILOV, V. et al.: 'Investigations of Chronic Gamma-Irradiation of the Heart, the Liver and the Kidneys'. *Neoplasma* 12 (1965) S. 305. – Ref. in: *Arch. f. Geschwulstforsch.* 27 (1966) Nr. 2, S. 185

MONOD, J.: 'Biosynthese eines Enzyms'. *Angewandte Chemie* 1959, Nr. 22

MONOD, J.: Molekularbiologische Aspekte des Krebsproblems. 'Der Mensch und die Technik' (*Techn. – Wuss.Bl. d. Südd. Z.*) 12 (26.2.70) Nr. 161

MORI, N.: 'Filtrierbare Vira und Krebs...' *Krebsarzt* 4 (1949) S. 309–313

MÖSE, J. R.: 'Versuche zu einer serologischen Tumordiagnostik mittels sporenbildender Bakterien'. *Z. Krebsforsch.* 73 (1970) S. 329–341

NAUTS, H. C., SWIFT, W. E. u. COLEY, B. L.: 'Treatment of Malignant Tumors by Bacterial Toxins...' *Cancer Res.* 6 (1946) S. 205–215

NAUTS, H. C., PELNER, L. u. FOWLER, G. A.: *Sarcoma of the Soft Tissues – other than Lymphosarcoma – Treated by Toxin-Therapy...* Cancer Research Institute, Inc., New York 1959

NEBEL, A.: *Berliner Homöop. Z.* 1914, Nr. 12 u. 1915, Nr. 6

NEBEL, A.: 'Aus meiner Krebsforschung und Krebsbehandlung'. In: SCHLEGEL, E.: *Die Krebskrankheit – ihre Natur und ihre Heilmittel.* (S. 263–282) Hippokrates-Verlag, Stuttgart, 2. Aufl. 1927

NEBEL, A.: 'Zur Methodik des Nachweises des Agens in malignen Tumoren'. *Krebsarzt* 3 (1948) S. 376–377

NEUBURGER-PAGEL: *Handbuch der Geschicht der Medizin.* 3 Bände. 1902–1905

NEUGEBAUER, H.: 'Nachweise für die Richtigkeit der ARNDT-SCHULZ-schen Heilregel'. *Allg. Hom. Ztg.* 199 (1954) Nr. 8, S. 253

NICHOLS, J. D. u. PRESLEY, J.: *Please Doctor Do Something.* Natural Food Associates, Atlanta, Texas 1972

NISSLE, A.: 'Über die Bedeutung der Dysbakterie des Colons für die Pathogenese des Krebses'. *Münch. Med. Wschr.* 95 (1953) S. 317–319

NOSSAL, G. J. V.: *Antibodies and Immunity.* Basic Books Inc., New York, N.Y. 1969

NOSSAL, G. J. V.: 'Immunologie und Krebs'. *Die Gelben Hefte* (Behring-Werke, Marburg/Lahn) 12 (1972) Nr. 1, S. 1–4

OBERLING, Ch.: *Krebs – Das Rätsel seiner Entstehung.* Rowohlt, Hamburg 1959

OLD, L. J. et al.: 'The Role of the Reticulo-Endothelial System in the Host Reaction to Neoplasia'. *Cancer Research* 21 (1961) Nr. 9, S. 1281–1300

OSWALD, W.: 'Krebs und Abwehr'. *Ars Medici* 59 (1969) Nr. 9, S. 608–619

OETTGEN, H. F. et al.: 'Tumorimmunologie'. *Dtsch. Med. Wschr.* 93 (1968) S. 1072 u. 1157

PAPANICOLAOU, G. N. u. TRAUT, H. F.: *Diagnosis of Uterine Cancer by the Vaginal Smear.* The Commonwealth Fund, New York 1943

PELNER, L. u. FOWLER, G. A.: 'Sarcoma of the Soft Tissues . . . Treated by Toxin Therapy'. *J. Amer. Geriatrics Soc.* 7 (1959) S. 624–647 u. 698–729

PICK, J.: 'Konstitutionell-immunbiologische Behandlung der Krebs-krankheit. *Hippokrates* 22 (1951) Nr. 5, S. 127–131

PISCHINGER, A.: 'Krebs und Abwehreinrichtungen des Organismus'. *Krebsarzt* 21 (1966) Nr. 5, S. 297–311

PISCHINGER, A.: 'Über das vegetative Grundsystem'. *Physik. Med. u. Rehabil.* 10 (1969) S. 53–57

PONCET, A. u. LÉRICHE, R.: *La Tuberculose inflammatoire.* Octave Doin & fils, Paris 1912

POTTENGER, F. M. u. SIMONSEN, D. G.: 'Heat Labile Factors Necessary for the Proper Growth and Development of Cats'. *J. Lab. & Clin. Med.* (St. Louis/USA) 25 (1939) Nr. 6

RECKEWEG, H. H.: 'Die wissenschaftlichen Grundlagen der biologischen Medizin'. *Homotoxin-Journal* 10 (1971) Nr. 6, S. 345–359

RICCABONA, A.: 'Die dentogene Kieferhöhlen-Affektion'. *Zahnärztl. Prax.* 13 (1966) S. 225; Jahresberichte d. DAH 14 (1965/66) S. 134

RICKER, G.: *Allgemeine Pathophysiologie als Beitrag für eine Grundlage der Theorie der Medizin von A.D. SPERANSKY.* Hippokrates-Verlag, Stuttgart 1948

RÖNTGEN, W. C.: *Grundlegende Abhandlungen über X-Strahlen.* C. Kabitzsch, Würzburg 1915

ROOS, B.: 'Makrophagen: Herkunft, Entwicklung, Funktion'. In: BÜCHNER-LETTERER-ROULER: *Handb. d. Allg. Pathologie.* Band VII/3, S. 1–128. Springer, Berlin 1970

RÖSSLE, R.: VIRCHOW's *Archiv* 288 (1930) 781

ROUS, P.: 'Virus Tumors and Tumor Problem'. *Amer. J. Cancer* 28 (1936) S. 233–272

RUBIN, A.: 'Human Resistance to Cancer. I. Prognosis in Pelvic Malignancy Correlation between Patient Survival and Tissue Culture Growth of Tumors'. *Amer. J. Obstet. Gynec.* 85 (1963) S. 149–155. – Ref. in: Excerpta Medica, Section 16: Cancer 11/11 (1963) S. 1074

RUSCH, H. P.: 'Die Normalflora, ein neues Kriterium für gesunde Lebens- und Heilweise'. *Heilkunst* 64 (1951) Nr. 1

RUSCH, V.: 'Wissenschaftliche Grundlagen der Symbiose-Lenkung als Therapie'. *Physik. Med. u. Rehab.* 13 (1972) S. 122–129

SALZBORN, E.: 'Zur Behandlung des inoperablen Carcinoms'. *Wien. Med. Wschr.* 1. April 1939

SAMUELS, J.: 'Über eine kausale Therapie des Krebses . . .' *Münch. Med. Wschr.* 96 (1954) Nr. 25, S. 724–726 u. 26, S. 756–759

SANDER, F. F.: *Der Säure-Basen-Haushalt des menschlichen Organismus.* Hippokrates-Verlag, Stuttgart 1953

SANTO, E.: 'Autogame Tumorgenese'. *Was gibt es Neues in der Medizin?* 4 (1952/53)

SANTO, E.: 'Die Reproduktion von Zellen des Typs weißer Blutkörperchen mit Hilfe von Coli-Bakterien'. *Medizin heute* 1956, Nr. 3

SCHADE, H.: *Die Molekular-Pathologie der Entzündung*. Th. Steinkopff, Dresden 1935

SCHEUERLEN: *Dtsch. Med. Wschr.* 1886, S. 48; 1887, S. 1033; 1888, S. 617; *Berliner Klin. Wschr.* 1887, S. 935.

SCHEURLEN, P. G.: 'Immunologische Aspekte bösartiger Tumoren'. *Med. Welt* 22 (1971) S. 1257–1261

SCHLEGEL, O.: 'Gedanken über die "Unheilbarkeit" des Krebses'. *Hippokrates* 26 (1955) Nr. 19, S. 573–577

SCHLIEPHAKE, E.: 'Behandlung mit künstlicher Überwärmung des Körpers'. *Jahreskurse f. ärztl. Fortb.* 33 (1942) Nr. 8

SCHLIEPHAKE, E.: 'Das Krebsproblem in neuer Beleuchtung'. *Hippokrates* 23 (1952) Nr. 16, S. 431–433

SCHLIEPHAKE, E.: 'Zur Technik der Auto-Hormon-Therapie mit Kurzwellen'. *Erfahrungsheilk.* 18 (1969) S. 37–40

SCHLÜREN, E. u. DÖBLER, S.: 'Ergebnisse in der Immuntherapie des Karzinoms'. *Krebsgeschehen* 1 (3) (1971) S. 125 (153) – 129 (157)

SCHMÄHL, D.: *Entstehung, Wachstum und Chemotherapie maligner Tumoren*. Editio Cantor KG., Aulendorg. 2. Aufl. 1970

SCHMID, F.: 'Mechanismen der körpereigenen Abwehr'. *Physik. Med. u. Rehab.* 9 (1968) S. 214–218

SCHOELER, H.: *Das Hochpotenz-Problem in der Homöopathie*. K. F. Haug, Saulgau 1951

SCHULTZ VAN TREECK, A.: 'Krebs und körpereigene Abwehr'. *Laryngologie* 33 (1954) Nr. 7/8

SCHWAMM, E.: 'Ultra-Rot-Strahlung und Krebsgeschehen'. *Erfahrungsheilk.* 3 (1954) S. 313–317

SEEGER, P. G.: 'Die Bedeutung einer umfassenden Prophylaxe des Krebses ...' *Wetter-Boden-Mensch* 1970, Nr. 9, S. 457–466

SELYE, H.: *Einführung in die Lehre vom Adaptationssyndrom*. G. Thieme, Stuttgart 1953

SIEGMUND, G.: 'Die Begründung der "Ganzheits-Medizin".' *Hippokrates* 25 (1954) Nr. 13, S. 397–400

SMITHERS, D. W.: *A Clinical Prospect of the Cancer Problem*. London u. Edinburgh 1960

SOUTHAM: 'The Immunologic State of Patients with Non-Lymphomatous Cancer'. *Cancer Res.* 28 (1968) S. 1433

SPENGLER, C.: *Tuberkulose- und Syphilis-Arbeiten*. H. Erfurt, Davos 1911

SPERANSKY, A. D.: *Grundlagen der Theorie der Medizin*. Dr. Saenger, Berlin 1950

STANDENATH: 'Grundprobleme der allgemeinen Pathologie und Therapie. – Entzündung und Fieber'. *Theorie u. Praxis in der Medizin* 4 (1935) S. 243, 298 u. 337, ferner 5 (1935) S. 5 u. 29

STANLEY, W. M.: 'Die Beziehungen zwischen Viren und Krebs'. *Krebsarzt* 12 (1957) Nr. 6, S. 307–320

STÖGER, R.: 'Gezielte interne Krebsbehandlung', *Med. Welt* 1967, S. 3183. – Ref. in: *Krebsarzt* 23 (1968) Nr. 4, S. 307

STROBL, A.: 'Die Zungendiagnostik als Hilfmittel des prakt. Arztes'. *Erfahrungsheilk*. 9957, Nr. 9; Sonderdruck d. K. F. Haug, Heidelberg

THIELEMANN, K.: 'Die Bedeutung der Gebiß-Sanierung. *Erfahrungsheilk*. 18 (1969) Nr. 7, S. 241–245

THOMAS, L.: In: LAWRENCE, H. S.: 'Cellular and Humoral Aspects of the Hypersensitive States'. (S. 529) (*Symposia of the Section on Microbiology, N.Y. Academy of Medicine*, Nr. 9) Cassel, London 1959

TREPEL, F.: 'Tumor-Antigene und Immun-Reaktionen gegen Tumoren'. *Med. Klin.* 66 (1971) S. 215–222

TREPEL, F.: 'Immunologische Tumor-Therapie'. *Med. Klin.* 66 (1971) S. 222–229

VEIL, W. H.: *Fokalinfektion und Bedeutung des Herdinfekts für die menschl. Pathologie*. G. Fischer, Jena 1940

VEIL, W. H. u. STURM, A.: *Die Pathologie des Stammhirns und ihre vegetativen klinischen Bilder*. G. Fischer, Jena 1942

VESTER, F.: 'Krebsforschung, ein Problem der Wissenschaftsstruktur'. (Neue Aspekte der Krebsforschung) Vortrag im Süddeutschen Rundfunk am 24.5.70

VILLEQUÉZ, E.: *Le parasitisme latent des cellules du sang chez l'homme, en particulier dans le sang des cancéreux*. Librairie Maloine, Paris 1955

VIRCHOW, R.: *Die Cellularpathologie*. A. Hirschwald, Berlin. 1. Aufl. 1858

VOLL, R.: *Medikament-Testung, Nosoden-Therapie und Mesenchym-Entschlackungs-Therapie bzw. Mesenchym-Reaktivierung*. Med. – Liter. Verlag, Uelzen 1960

VOLL, R.: *Wechselbeziehungen von odontogenen Herden zu Organen und Gewebssystemen*. Med. – Lit. Verlag, Uelzen, 2. Aufl. 1970

WARBURG, O.: *Über den Stoffwechsel der Tumoren*. Springer, Berlin 1926

WARNING, H.: 'Die Ernährungsfrage und die Bedeutung der POTTENGERschen Katzenversuche'. *Hippokrates* 25 (1954) Nr. 24, S. 761–763

WARNING, H.: 'Gift in der Luft'. *Diaita* 5 (1959) Nr. 1, S. 5–9

WEHRLI, F.: 'Die Hämatogene Oxydations-Therapie'. (H-O-T) *Medizin heute* 7 (1958) S. 97–106

WERTH, G.: 'Malignolipin'. *Med. Welt* 21 (1970) Nr. 36, S. 1547–1553

WINDSTOSSER, K.: 'Der ENDERLEIN-sche Endobiont – 30 Jahre Bakterien-Cyklogenie'. *Erfahrungsheilk.* 6 (1957) Nr. 1

WINDSTOSSER, K.: 'Ganzheitsmedizinische Diagnostik und Therapie der dentalen Herderkrankungen'. *Das Dtsch. Zahnärzteblatt* 1958, Nr. 1/2

WINSDTOSSER, K.: 'Aktiviertes Autohämolysat zur verbesserten Eigenblutbehandlung'. *Physik.-Diätetische Therapie* 5 (1964) Nr. 11

WOLF, M. u. RANSBERGER, K.: *Enzymtherapie*. W. Maudrich, Wien 1970

WOLFF, J.: *Die Lehre von der Krebskrankheit*. 4 Bände. G. Fischer, Jena. 1. Aufl. 1907–1928 (1. Bd. 1906/07, 2. Bd. 1911, 3. Bd. 1913/14, 4. Bd. 1928) u. 2. Aufl. 1929 (1. Bd.)

WRBA, H.: 'Der gegenwärtige Stand der Krebsforschung'. *Krebsarzt* 23 (1968) Nr. 2, S. 83–90

ZABEL, W.: *Ganzheitsbehandlung der Geschwulsterkrankungen*. (Bericht über den 5. Berchtesgadener Kurs für Ganzheitsmedizin, Okt. 1952) Hippokrates-Verlag, Stuttgart 1953

ZABEL, W.: *Körpereigene Abwehr gegen Krebs?* Med. – Lit. Verlag, Hamburg 1964

ZABEL, W.: *Die interne Krebstherapie und die Ernährung des Krebskranken*. Bircher-Benner-Verlag, Bad Homburg v.d.H. 1968

ZADIK, P.: 'Über das Prinzip allgemeiner und ... spezieller Krebsverhütung ...' *Krebsarzt* 22 (1967) S. 251–261

ZILBER, L. A.: 'Die Virustheorie der Geschwulstentstehung'. Nowotwory 11 (1961) S. 249. – Ref. in: *Arch. f. Geschwulstforsch.* 20 (1962) Nr. 1, S. 46

THIRD OPINION—FOURTH EDITION

An International Directory to Alternative Therapy Centers for the Treatment and Prevention of Cancer & Other Degenerative Diseases

John M. Fink

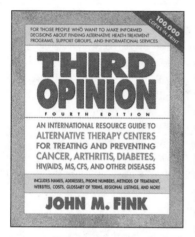

In an age of information, when there is a growing awareness and acceptance of the value of alternative and complementary medicine, it's surprising that basic facts about alternative cancer treatments are so hard to come by. If you don't know the right person, it may take days or even weeks to learn even the simplest of facts. Worse, sometimes information becomes available only as a matter of chance.

Here, in this fourth revised edition, is a comprehensive guide to the growing number of alternative treatment centers located throughout the world. Everything you need to know—from addresses, phone numbers, names, and prices, to philosophical approaches and methods of treatment—is provided in a clear, easy-to-use format. Also included are the educational centers, information services, and support programs that may be of interest to the person looking for alternative or adjunctive therapy. For each listing, the author has gathered all of the information necessary to make that all-important initial contact. To further help you, the author has included a glossary of terms, a regional breakdown of centers, and a list of informative readings.

Beyond any first and second opinions that may be offered, there are other options that you may wish to consider. *Third Opinion* offers you the opportunity to learn about these options so that you can make a truly informed decision.

John M. Fink had been an actor for fourteen years when he lost his young daughter to cancer. Since then, he has been deeply interested in alternative and adjunctive care. He has been active as a board member of the International Association of Cancer Victors and Friends, both nationally and in the Santa Barbara Chapter. He has also been on the Board of the National Health Federation, and has served as a member of the Advisory Panel for the Congressional Office of Technology Assessment's (OTA) study, Unconventional Cancer Treatments. He resides in southern California with his wife.

$19.95 • 382 pages • 7.5 x 9-inch paperback • ISBN 0-7570-0131-9

RETHINKING CANCER

Non-Traditional Approaches to the Theories, Treatments, and Prevention of Cancer

Ruth Sackman

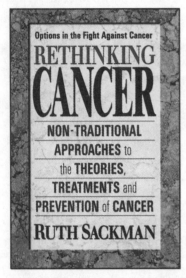

For over thirty years, the Foundation for Advancement in Cancer Therapy (FACT) has acted as a consumer advocacy group, educating cancer patients about alternative therapies and their rights as patients. Although traditional medical groups have often ignored or disregarded the groundbreaking work of complementary medical researchers, FACT has provided these pioneers with a platform to be heard. The foundation's intention has never been to discredit conventional medicine, but rather to scrutinize alternative therapies and enable cancer patients and their families to make informed decisions regarding treatment options.

Unfortunately, there still remains a major gap in the distribution of information on noninvasive treatments. To meet this challenge, Ruth Sackman, cofounder and President of FACT, has written *Rethinking Cancer*. Here, you'll find pertinent information on a wide variety of topics, including the major role of nutrition in health, the methods available to repair the body's biological breakdowns, and strategies for achieving detoxification. The author provides valid research and offers specific advice on treating the body as a whole, rather than treating just the cancer.

Ruth Sackman is the cofounder and president of the Foundation for Advancement in Cancer Therapy (FACT), a thirty-year old consumer advocacy organization that provides information on alternative cancer therapies. Based in New York City, Ms. Sackman has dedicated her life to the pursuit of nontoxic approaches to the treatment of cancer.

$16.95 • 248 pages • 6 x 9-inch paperback • ISBN 0-7570-0093-2

RECOVERY FROM CANCER

The Remarkable Story of One Woman's Struggle With Cancer & What She Did to Beat the Odds

Ruth Sackman

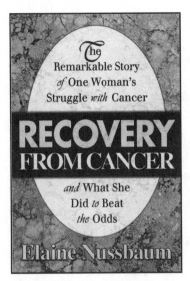

The words slowly sank in—
Mrs. Nussbaum, you have cancer.
So began Elaine Nussbaum's very personal struggle with this frightening disease. Despite surgery, chemotherapy, and radiation, Elaine's cancer spread to her bones and both lungs. Three years after her initial diagnosis, she had had enough of conventional therapies. Elaine stopped all medications and treatments, and began to practice macrobiotics in a last-ditch effort to save her life. Slowly, her condition improved. Steadily, she regained her health. As Elaine recovered from the ravages of cancer, her family drew upon her newly found strength to become whole once again.

Here, then, in Elaine's own words, is her inspiring story of recovery against all odds—from her first days in the hospital, to the agony reflected in the faces of her family, to her eventual triumph.

Elaine's dramatic and very moving story offers hope to cancer patients everywhere—and adds to the growing evidence that macrobiotics can be effective in the treatment of this insidious disease.

Elaine Nussbaum holds a bachelor's degree in business education from Montclair State College. After her painful experience with cancer, she became a professional nutritionist and certified teacher of macrobiotics. Elaine has now been practicing, studying, and teaching macrobiotics for almost a decade. She has an active consulting practice in West Orange, New Jersey, and also offers macrobiotic cooking classes.

Elaine is a popular lecturer, having spoken to groups throughout the United States. She has also been interviewed on numerous radio and national television shows. Elaine and her husband, Ralph, currently reside in northern New Jersey.

$16.95 • 192 pages • 6 x 9-inch paperback • ISBN 0-7570-0137-8

CONFESSIONS OF A KAMIKAZE COWBOY

A True Story of Discovery, Acting, Health, Illness, Recovery, and Life

Dirk Benedict

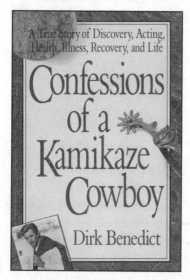

Initially, *Confessions of a Kamikaze Cowboy* tells the fascinating story of Dirk Benedict's journey from the big sky country of Montana to the hustle and hype of Hollywood. It also vividly describes his personal odyssey of self-exploration, discovery, and growth—from struggling actor to celebrity, from meat eater to vegetarian, from cancer victim to cancer victor.

Confessions of a Kamikaze Cowboy is brilliantly written—insightful, witty, humorous, and always challenging. While you may not agree with everything this book has to say, it will make you reconsider a great many truths in your own life.

Dirk Benedict has starred on Broadway, in films, and in several hit television series, including *The A Team* and *Battlestar Galactica*. When he's not making a movie or writing screenplays, he pilots his own airplane, composes music, plays the piano and trombone, goes fishing, or just relaxes with his two sons. Dirk Benedict divides his time between California and Montana.

$14.95 • 232 pages • 6 x 9-inch paperback • ISBN 0-7570-0277-3